COMPLETE CDM KEY

Copyright © June 2023 **COMPLETE CDM KEY**

All rights are reversed. Except as permitted under the United States Copyright Act 1976, no part of this publication can be reproduced or distributed in any form or by any means, or stored in a database or retrieved system. Without the prior written permission from the Author.

Terms of use

This book named COMPLETE CDM KEY is a copyrighted eBook and it's licensors reserve all rights and to the work. Use of this book is subject to these terms.

COMPLETE CDM KEY

CHAPTER 3	
CARDIOLOGY	3
CHAPTER	45
RESPIRATORY	45
CHAPTER	87
GASTROENTEROLOGY	87
Chapter	160
RENAL AND GENITOURINARY	160
CHAPTER	180
ENDOCRINOLOGY	180
CHAPTER	200
NEUROLOGY	200
CHAPTER	222
RHEUMATOLOGY	222
CHAPTER	253
DERMATOLOGY	253
CHAPTER	267
OBSTETRICS AND GYNAECOLOGY	267
CHAPTER	277
PAEDIATRICS	277
CHAPTER	337
PSYCHIATRY	337
PRACTICE PAPER	365
REFERENCES	403

CHAPTER

CARDIOLOGY

CASE 1

SCENARIO

A 35 years old woman who first presented to the office for biliary colic now has had an elevated serum cholesterol level on 3 separate tests. Family history reveals that his 60 years old mother recently had a MI and that his 66 years old father has T2DM. The patient does not smoke but drinks beer and wine moderately, and he regularly has caffeinated soft drinks with his meals. He experiences periodic stress related to his occupation.

Lab results are as follows:

Urinalysis - normal

Complete book count - normal

Blood Glucose - normal

Triglycerides - 3.2

Total Cholesterol - 6.2

Cholesterol, LDL - 3.40

HDL - 0.9

What will you advise this patient to do to from following recommendations, select all appropriate.

1. A diet in which 20% of calories come from saturated fats.

COMPLETE CDM KEY

2. A diet in which total fat intake is less than 30% of calories.

3. A new occupation.

4. 3-hydroxyl-3-methyl-CoA (HMG-CoA) reductase inhibitors.

5. Benzphetamine.

6. Stop all dairy products.

7. Elimination of beer but allowance red wine.

8. Gastric bypass.

9. Increase physical activity.

10. Laxatives.

11. Fibric acid derivatives.

12. Phentermine.

13. Nicotinic acid.

14. No recommendations

15. A diet that provides less than 300 mg cholesterol each day.

CASE 2

SCENARIO

A 50-year-old man had a myocardial infarction and was taken to hospital. During his admission, he developed symptoms of left ventricular systolic dysfunction.

01   List 2 symptoms of left ventricular systolic dysfunction (LVSD).

_____

_____

02   Name 4 chest X-ray findings that you would expect to see in LVSD.

COMPLETE CDM KEY

03 Your consultant asks you to arrange and echocardiogram. He asks you what features you expect to see on the echo?

The patient is admitted to the coronary care unit. Whilst updating the patient's family, you try to remember the pathophysiology of heart failure.

04 Give 2 compensatory mechanisms involved in trying to maintain cardiac output.

05 What are preload and after-load?

COMPLETE CDM KEY

06 Define Starling's law.

_____
_____
_____
_____

The management plan for this patient includes administering furosemide.

07 Why does the administration of furosemide require regular blood tests?

_____
_____
_____
_____

08 Name 2 lifestyle modifications that should be considered as part of the patient's management.

_____
_____
_____
_____

COMPLETE CDM KEY

CASE 3

SCENARIO

A 76-year-old man presents to the A&E department with sudden onset, central crushing chest pain. He is nauseated and sweating profusely. The patient's electrocardiogram shows ST elevation in loads $V_2 - V_5$ and you therefore make a diagnosis of anterior myocardial infarction.

01 What pathophysiological process has taken place in the coronary artery to cause the myocardial infarction?

02 Which coronary artery is most likely to be affected?

03 You are in a rural district general hospital. List 2 fibrinolytic drugs that you would consider.

COMPLETE CDM KEY

The patient is subsequently found to have severe three vessel coronary artery disease. He later undergoes coronary artery bypass grafting (CABG)

04   What vessels may be used as grafts in CABG?

A few days later the patient develops a post-operation pyrexia (38.2 'C).

05   List 3 potential causes of the pyrexia.

COMPLETE CDM KEY

CASE 4

SCENARIO

You are the on-call FY2 when a 70-year-old woman is admitted with sudden dyspnea. She denies any pain and she apyrexial. She is a heavy smoker.

01 Name 6 features from the patient's history that you would enquire about to narrow down the cause of her breathlessness.

_____
_____
_____
_____
_____
_____

You examine her cardiovascular system thoroughly and discover that she has an ejection systolic murmur. You decide this may be secondary to aortic stenosis.

02 List 4 other examination features that would be in keeping with aortic stenosis.

COMPLETE CDM KEY

03 Whilst you try to arrange an echo, you ask the FY1 to do an ECG. What do you expect to see on the ECG?

04 An echo is subsequently performed. What would you want to know from the echo and why?

CASE 5

SCENARIO:

A 76 years old woman comes to the office for a blood pressure check. She recently returned from her annual 6 months stay in Miami. You observe several lesions on her forehead and cheek. You ask her about the lesions and she says, they don't bother her.

What will you advise this patient to do to prevent further similar lesions?

CASE 6

SCENARIO

A 62-year-old woman presents to A&E with crushing chest pain which radiates down her left arm. She looks grey and unwell. You think she may be having a myocardial infarction.

01 Give 2 other diagnostic criteria that would support your diagnosis.

02 Investigations confirm that your patient is having an MI. your consultant decides that thrombolysis is in her best interests. He asks if you can name 3 contraindications to thrombolysis?

COMPLETE CDM KEY

COMPLETE CDM KEY

03 She makes makes a good recovery and eventually she is ready for discharge. She was already on aspirin. Excluding this, give 3 classes of drugs that she should be discharged on and briefly explain their mechanisms of action.

04 Describe 4 lifestyle modifications that you would encourage in your patient.

CASE 7

SCENARIO

A 43-year-old man presents to the A&E department with symptoms of left ventricular failure.

01 List 2 symptoms of left heart failure.

_____

_____

02 Which initial radiological investigation above that you would expect to see in a patient with LVF.

_____

_____

In A&E the FY2 gives the patient 5mg IV morphine to relieve their distress. When you arrive in A&E, you examine the patient and find an irregular pulse. An ECG confirms atrial fibrillation. The patient says the felt palpitations acutely in the last few hours.

COMPLETE CDM KEY

03 List 2 drugs that you would prescribe in this circumstance. What does would you prescribe? Describe their mechanism of action.

04 The patient is hypotensive. Which route of administration would you use and why?

CASE 8

SCENARIO

You are an FY2 doing a rotation in general practice. A 60-year-old man has come to see you. His blood pressure is 154 systolic, 96 phase 5 diastolic.

01   What is phase 5 in relation to BP?.

02   Give 2 examples of your next course of action regarding his BP.

The patient's BP remains high on several occasions. You decide he has needs treatment. However, because he is asymptomatic he really isn't keen on drug treatment.

03   Suggest 2 long-term advantages of good BP control.

COMPLETE CDM KEY

04 Suggest 3 classes of drugs that could be used in hypertension.

The patient is still anxious about long-term medication. He has lots of question and asks you about the side-effects of the drugs you suggested.

05. List 1 common side-effect for each class of drug in your answer to Question 4.

COMPLETE CDM KEY

COMPLETE CDM KEY

CASE 9

SCENARIO

An 82-year-old man complains of having leg pain at night. He smokes 50 cigarettes per day.

01 You think he has peripheral vascular disease (PVD). Give 3 features you would expect to find in the history which would support your diagnosis.

02 Give 4 features you would look for on examination.

03   List 3 investigations you would consider

CASE 10

SCENARIO

An 76-year-old man presents to A&E with severe shortness of breath. When you examine him, you find that he has a raised jugular venous pressure and crackles at the lung bases.

01   What is the significance of raised JVP and crackles at the lung bases?

02   Your management plan includes the administration of a diuretic. Which class would you use and why?

COMPLETE CDM KEY

The patient subsequently developed diuretic-induced hypokalemia and so you give spironolactone to prevent this.

03 Name 1 other drug that has a similar effect.

COMPLETE CDM KEY

04   What are the other benefits of using spironolactone in a case like this?

05   The cardiologist considered, but then discounted using digoxin, bisoprolol and dobutamine. Give 1 reason for rejecting each of these.

The patient was started on an ACE inhibitor.

06   Name 2 precautionary measures that should be undertaken before starting an ACE inhibitor.

CASE 11

SCENARIO

You are the FY1 on your first night shift covering all the medical patients in a large district general hospital. You are paged by one of the nurses from coronary care who asks you to come urgently to assess a 70-year-old woman with a history of heart failure. When you examine her, you find her to be extremely unwell, with a respiratory rate of 40 and widespread crepitations in both lungs. You diagnose acute pulmonary oedema.

01 What is your immediate management plan?

02 You arrange a beside chest X-ray. What appearances would support your diagnosis?

COMPLETE CDM KEY

03 When you reassess the patient, you hear a pansystolic murmur at the apex. What is likely to be responsible for this?

_____

_____

04 The patient has had mild heart failure for years. Suggest 3 possible causes for her acute deterioration.

_____

_____

_____

_____

_____

_____

CASE 12

SCENARIO

A 64-years-old man presents complaining of lethargy and night sweats. He appears unwell and is febrile. When you auscultate the heart, you hear a soft systolic murmur. You suspect infective endocarditis.

01   What other clinical signs would support your suspicion?

02   What investigations would you request to support your diagnosis?

03   Give other causes of pyrexia of unknown origin (PUO).

CASE 13

SCENARIO

You are the FY2 working in A&E. You assess a 50-year-old Asian man who smokes 20 cigarettes a day. He describes several months' history of exertional chest pain radiating into his neck.

01   Name 4 risk factors for developing coronary artery disease (CAD).

You decide to admit the patient because he has ongoing pain. Investigations exclude myocardial infarction and he is diagnosed with angina.

02   List 4 potentially beneficial drugs that he could be started on and give a reason for prescribing each.

COMPLETE CDM KEY

COMPLETE CDM KEY

03 List 2 pathological ECG features in the anterior chest leads of an acute full thickness anterior myocardial infarction. Outline their electrophysiological cause.

CARDIOLOGY

ANSWERS

CASE 1

1. A diet that provides less than 300 mg of cholesterol each day

2. Increase physical activity

3. A diet in which total fat intake is less than 30% of calories

Case 2: Myocardial infarction

01. **Symptoms of left ventricular systolic dysfunction (LVSD) include:**

- Orthopnoea
- Paroxysmal nocturnal dyspnoea
- Nocturnal cough (with frothy, pink spit)
- Nocturia
- Poor exercise tolerance
- Fatigue

02. **CXR findings in keeping with LVSD include (think ABCDE):**

- Signs of aveolar pulmonary oedema (e.g. bat's wings appearance of lung fields adjacent to hila, fluffy opacity of lung fields)
- Signs of interstitial pulmonary oedema (e.g. Karley B lines, fluid in the horizontal fissure)
- Cardiomegaly (>1/2 thoracic diameter)
- Dilated upper lobe vessels (upper lobe diversion)
- Pleural effusion (usually bilateral)

03. **Echo findings in LVSD:**

- Signs of left ventricular dysfunction, e.g. non-compliant LV, LV dilatation of hypertrophy.
- Complications of MI that may have caused LVSD.
  - Aneurysm of myocardial wall
  - Mitral valve prolapse / rupture of chordae tendineae.
  - Rupture of ventricular septum
- Blood flow: poor LV ejection fraction (<40%), increased end-diastolic volume and stroke volume (EDV:SV)

04. **Compensatory mechanisms in LVSD:**

- Automatic: increased sympathetic activation (increases heart rate to maintain cardiac output)
- Renin-angiotensin-aldosterone system (RAAS): activated to increase BP and vasoconstriction.
- ADH: reduces urine output to retain water and thereof raises BP

05.

- **Preload** is the filling pressure of the heart (determined by venous return) which is applied to the myocardium.
- **Afterload** is the pressure against which the heat is pumping to eject blood (determined by total peripheral resistance)

06. **Starling's law:** the greater the stretch on the myocardium during diastole, the greater the subsequent stroke volume in systole.

07. **Monitor renal function whilst on furosemide because:** furosemide can cause renal impairment, hyponatraemia, hypokalaemia and hypocalcaemia.

08. **Life style modification in heart disease:**

- Smoking cessation.
- Weight loss
- Died low in saturated fat/cholesterol/salt
- Take up moderate exercise
- Reduce caffeine intake
- Reduce alcohol

Case 3: Anterior myocardial infarction

01. **Pathology of myocardial infarction:**

    - Atherosclerotic plaque rupture within a coronary artery leads to platelet aggregation and activation of the clotting cascade, resulting in thrombus formation and vessel narrowing / occlusion.
    - This interruption of blood flow to the myocardium can be severe or total, and leads to myocardial ischaemia and nerosis (ST elevation)

02. **Anterior STEMI:** left main stem / left coronary artery As ST elevation is seen across both the anteroseptal and lateral areas of the heart, this indicates an occlusion in the left coronary artery before it splits into the left anterior descending and the circumflex artery.

03. **Fibrinolytics:**

    - Alteplase (rtPA)
    - Tenecteplase
    - Streptokinase

04. **Vessels in CABG:**

    - Internal mammary artery (Internal thoracic artery)
    - Long saphenous vein
    - Radial artery

05. **Causes of pyrexia:**

    - Wound infection at site of surgery
    - IV-line phlebitis
    - Pneumonia / lower respiratory tract infection
    - UTI
    - Endocarditis (from septicaemia secondary to surgery)
    - Pulmonary embolus / deep vein thrombosis.

COMPLETE CDM KEY

Case 4: Aortic stenosis

01. **Dyspnoea history:**

    - Onset: when did it come on, how suddenly, what was she doing at the time?
    - Duration: how long has she been breathless for?
    - Course: persistent or intermittent?
    - Progression: getting worse?
    - Severity: how breathless is she-can she talk in complete sentences, walk, is she breathless at rest?
    - Associated symptoms: cough, sputum, pain, haemoptysis
    - Features of breathlessness: is breathlessness worse when lying flat? Does she wake up during the night gasping for breath (PND)?
    - Exacerbating / relieving factors: provoked by exercise, cold air etc.

02. **Examination findings of aortic stenosis:**

    - Slow rising, flow volume pulse
    - Having, non-displaced apex beat
    - Thrill in aortic area?
    - Ejection systolic murmur, best heard at aortic area radiating to the carotids
    - Features of associated heart failure, e.g. fine basal crepitations
    - Narrow pulse pressure

03. **ECG features in aortic stenosis:**

    - Features of left ventricular hypertrophy with strain pattern
    - Left bundle branch block or complete heart block
    - P-mitrale

04. **Echo features of aortic stenosis:**

    - Saverity of aortic stenosis (severe if valve orifice <0.5cm^2)
    - Pressure gradient across the valve (severe if >50mmHg)

- Left ventricular hypertrophy, compliance and function: specifically end-diastolic volume (high if systolic dysfunction) and ejection fraction
- Other associated valve disease, e.g. co-existing regurgitation of aortic valve or disease of other valves
- These factors are important to know as they have prognostic implications
- The changes would be important in influencing whether surgery would be appropriate or not and can predict future complications

Case 5:

Decrease sun exposure and apply sunscreen; unblock; UV protection; avoiding tanning etc.

Case 6: Myocardial infarction

01. **Diagnostic criteria of MI:**
    - ECG changes – ST elevation, ST depression, pathological Q waves
    - Raised cardiac troponin (levels and timings vary depending on local labs)

02. **Absolute contraindications to thrombolysis:**
    - Previous intracranial haemorrhage
    - Known structural cerebral vascular lesion
    - Known malignant intracranial neoplasm
    - Ischaemic stroke within 3 months
    - Suspected aortic dissection
    - Active bleeding (excluding menses)
    - Significant closed head trauma or facial trauma within 3 months
    - Intracranial or intraspinal surgery within 2 months

COMPLETE CDM KEY

- Severe uncontrolled hypertension (unresponsive to emergency treatment)

COMPLETE CDM KEY

03. **Drugs post-MI:**

- Statins (e.g. atorvastatin): inhibit HMG CoA-reductase to reduce cholesterol formation and increase hepatic LDL receptor production leads to decreased serum LDL levels and decreased LDL uptake by the vascular endothelium which slows the progression of atherosclerotic plaques
- B-blockers (e.g. bisoprolol): antagonistic effect on adrenaline at B-adrenoreceptors, therefore reducing sympathetic drive on the heart resulting in a lowered heart rate.
- ACE inhibitors (e.g. ramipril): inhibit conversion of angiotensinogen to angiotensin I, therefore decrease angiotensin II and aldosterone production; this prevents angiotensin II mediated vasoconstriction and therefore reduces blood pressure.

04. **Life style modifications:**

- Weight reduction
- Regular daily exercise
- Diet low in salt, saturated fats and triglycerides
- Diet rich in oily fish, fruit, vegetables and fibre
- Smoking cessation

Case 7: Atrial fibrillation

01. **Symptoms of LVF:**

    - Dyspnoea (and associated orthopnoea and PND)
    - Lethargy and malaise
    - Cardiac wheeze / cough
    - Nocturia

02. **Chest X-ray would confirm pulmonary oedema**

03. **X-ray features of LVF:**

    - $\underline{A}$lveolar oedema
    - Kerley $\underline{B}$ lines
    - $\underline{C}$ardiomegaly
    - $\underline{D}$ilated upper lobe vessels
    - Pleural $\underline{e}$ffusion

04. **Pharmacological management of this patient:**

    - Amiodarone (used in reversible / acute AF):
        - 300mg IV over 20-30min then 900mg/24h via central line
        - Class III anti-arrhythmic: blocks K^+ channels, NA^+ channels, and B-adrenergic receptors to increase the duration of myocardial contraction in the atria and ventricles
        - This therefore reduces heart rate and vascular resistance Low
    - Low molecular weight heparin (LMWH)
        - Enoxaparin 1mg/kg twice daily SC unless active bleeding or high risk of bleeding
        - Binds to and enhances antithrombin III, which inhibits factor Xa therefore preventing thrombosis.
    - Furosemide
        - Inhibits tubular reabsorption of sodium and chloride in the proximal and distal tubules, as well as in the thick ascending loop of Henle by inhibiting sodium-chloride co-transport system resulting in excessive excretion of water along with sodium, chloride, magnesium and calcium.

05.
- Intravenous route
- Low blood pressure means the gut will be under-perfused and medication given orally will be poorly absorbed and metabolised, therefore intravenous administration provides greater bioavailability.

Case 8: Hypertension

01. Phase 5: The 5th Korotkoff sound: the phase at which heart sounds disappear as the cuff is deflating below the diastolic pressure

02. Initial management in this case:
- Take further readings after allowing him to relax and organize a return appointment in 2 weeks
- Take a history to assess risk factors and offer lifestyle advice

03. Advantages of good BP control:
- Reduce risk of cardiovascular events:
  - Stroke
  - Myocardial infarction
- Reduce risk of end-organ damage:
  - Renal impairment which may in the long term lead to need for renal replacement therapy
  - Hypertensive retinopathy which may lead to visual loss

COMPLETE CDM KEY

04. **Classes of antihypertensives:**

    - ACE inhibitor
    - Low molecular weight heparin (LMWH)
      - Dry cough
      - Postural hypotension
      - Hyperkalaemia
      - Renal failure
      - Angioedema
    - Thiazide diuretic:
      - Polyuria / nocturia
      - Hyponatraemia
      - Hypokalaemia
      - Gout
    - Calcium channel blocker:
      - Constipation
      - Headache, flushing
      - Fatigue
      - Gum hyperplasia
      - Ankle oedema

Case 9: Peripheral vascular disease

01. **Symptoms of PVD:**

    - Pain relieved by hanging feet out of bed / sleeping in chair at night
    - Pain provoked by walking and relieved by rest-intermittent claudication
    - Presence of risk factors: smoking, diabetes mellitus, obesity, family history
    - Past medical history: angina, myocardial infarction or stroke.

COMPLETE CDM KEY

02. **Examination features of PVD:**

    - Gangrene / ulceration (punched-out arterial ulcers of sloughy venous ulcers on gaiter area
    - Hypertrophic nails
    - Lipodermatosclerosis
    - Haemosiderin deposits
    - Shiny, atrophic skin
    - Hair loss
    - Varicose eczema
    - Absent pulses
    - Femoral bruit
    - Cold, white legs
    - Postural colour change (positive Buerger's test)

03. **Investigations in PVD:**

    - Blood: FBC, ESR/CRP (rule out arteritis), U&Es, lipids
    - ECG-exclude AF and assess suitability for possible surger
    - Ankle brachial pressure index (ABPI)
    - Colour duplex ultrasound
    - CT/MR angiogram of pelvis and legs.

Case 10: Pulmonary oedema

01. **Significance of raised JVP crackles:**

    - Raised JVP signifies right heart failure and crackles at lung bases are signs of pulmonary oedema secondary to left heart failure
    - Together this supports a clinical diagnosis of heart failure

02. **Loop diuretic:**

    - More potent diuretic action than thiazide or potassium –sparing diuretics
    - Faster onset of action
    - Is a vasodilator which therefore reduces preload

COMPLETE CDM KEY

03. **Potassium-sparing diuretics:**

    - Eplerenone
    - Triamterene
    - Amiloride hydrochloride

04. **Benefits of spironolactone:**

    - Reduce mortality by 30% when used with conventional therapy (RALES trial)
    - Improves endothelial function
    - Reduces ventricular remodelling

05.
    - Digoxin
        - Used for heart failure which has not responded to first-line diuretic therapy
        - Has a narrow therapeutic range so may be toxic if not carefully controlled
        - Only indicated for first-line therapy of heart failure if patient in AF
    - B-blockers:
        - Slow the heart rate and myocardial workload so will reduce the ejection fraction-because this is already low then it may worsen heart failure
    - Dobutamine:
        - Inotrope which increase myocardial O_2 demand-used temporarily for severe acute heart failure when other measures have failed under specialist advice

06. **Before starting an ACE inhibitor:**

    - Check for contraindications to ACE inhibitors, e.g. bilateral renal artery stenosis, hypotension, renal failure, electrolyte disturbances,
    - Monitor U&Es after starting drug

- Warn of side-effects, e.g. dry cough, taste disturbance, first does hypotension

Case 11: Acute pulmonary oedema

01. **Immediate management of pulmonary oedema and LVSD:** as with every acutely unwell patient… assess ABCE!

    - Sit patient up and give high flow oxygen
    - Morphine (2.5-5mg IV)-useful in agitation and for vasodilation
    - Furosemide (40-80mg IV)-higher doses may be required
    - Urinary catheter-monitor fluid balance
    - If not hypotensive, give GTN spray (2 puffs)
    - Consider nitrate infusion (2-10mg/h) if systolic BP 100mmHg

02. **CXR features in LVSD:**

    - Alveolar oedema
    - Kerley B lines
    - Cardiomegaly
    - Dilated upper lobe vessels (upper lobe diversion)
    - Pleural effusions

03. **Pansystolic murmur at apex**

    - Mitral regurgitation – maximal at the apex and often in late systole; transmitted to the axilla

04. **Potential causes of cardiac decompensation:**

    - Bacterial endocarditis causing new valvular regurgitation
    - Post-MI papillary muscle rupture and mitral regurgitation
    - Fluid overload
    - Co-existing infection, e.g. pneumonia, URTI
    - Pulmonary embolism
    - Arrhythmia
    - Malignant hypertension

Case 12: Pyrexia of unknown origin

01. **Clinical signs of infective endocarditis:** remember… fever + new murmur = infective endocarditis, until proven otherwise.

    - Splinter haemorrhages
    - Osler's nodes (painful, erythematous nodules)
    - Janeway lesions (flat, painless erythematous lesions on palms and soles)
    - Finger clubbing
    - Roth's spots
    - Petechiae
    - Splenomegaly

02. **Investigation in infective endocarditis:** Diagnosis is based on

    Duke criteria

    - Blood cultures (from 3 different sites)
    - Bloods: FBC, U&Es, CRP/ESR, LFTs, rheumatoid factor
    - Urinalysis (for microscopic haematuria)
    - Echocardiogram (look for vegetations)
    - ECG (look for heart block)
    - Chest X-ray (cardiomegaly, pulmonary oedema)
    - CT (to look for emboli)

03. **Causes of PUO:**

    - Infection (20-40%): pyogenic abscess, TB, IE, primary HIV infection
    - Malignant disease (10-30%): lymphoma, leukaemia, renal cell carcinoma, hepatocellular carcinoma
    - Vasculitides (15-25%): rheumatoid arthritis, systemic lupus erythematosus, temporal cell arteritis
    - Miscellaneous (10-25%): drug fevers, thyrotoxicosis, inflammatory bowel disease, sarcoid
    - Pulmonary embolism, MI
    - Idiopathic / undiagnosed causes (5-25%):

Case 13: Coronary artery disease

01. **CAD risk factors:**

    - Hypertension
    - Smoking
    - High cholesterol
    - Male sex
    - Obesity
    - Diabetes
    - Stress
    - Family history

02. **Drug in CAD:**

    - **ACE inhibitor** (e.g. rampiril):
      - Reduces blood pressure via inhibition of renin-aldosterone-angiotensin system (RAAS), improving mortality (as hypertension is a risk factor for stroke and MI)
    - **Statin** (e.g. simvastatin):
      - Lowers cholesterol which therefore reduces the progression of atherosclerosis and decreases the risk of a cardiovascular event
    - **β-blocker** (e.g. atenolol):
      - Improves symptoms and reduces mortality by slowing heart rate
    - **Antiplatelet therapy** (e.g. aspirin):
      - Inhibits thromboxane A_2 to prevent platelet aggregation, therefore reducing the risk of thrombus formation
    - **GTN spray:**
      - Provides pain relief by temporarily causing myocardial vasodilation

03. **ECG changes in acute anterior STEMI:**

    - **ST elevation:** current from injury in myocardium leads to abnormal repolarisation of ventricular tissue; this causes ST segment elevation of $\geq$ 2mm in 2 or more contiguous chest leads as this portion corresponds to the time between ventricular depolarisation and repolarisation
    - **Q waves:** a 'window' effect is created where there is decreased conduction in the infarcted ventricle so the chest lead 'sees

through' the myocardium on the other side of the heart where the current is travelling away from the lead.

CHAPTER

RESPIRATORY

CASE 1

SCENARIO

You assess a 69-year-old woman with frequent lower respiratory tract infections and increasing shortness of breath. She smokes 40 cigrates per day. You think she may have COPD.

COMPLETE CDM KEY

01. Name 2 diseases that are found in patients with COPD.

02. Give 2 pathophysiological features of the diseases from your answer above.

03. Name 3 investigations you would request, and describe what results you would expect in a patient with COPD.

COMPLETE CDM KEY

04. The most common cause of COPD in the Western world is smoking. Name 4 methods that may help your patient stop smoking.

The patient improves from their infective exacerbation of COPD. You see her back in the respiratory clinic and she has successfully given up smoking and now enjoys vaping. You decide to prescribe her some inhalers.

05. Suggest 2 inhalers that may be beneficial and describe their mechanism of action.

COMPLETE CDM KEY

RESPIRATORY

CASE 2

SCENARIO

A 64-year-old woman with a history of COPD presents with cough and increased shortness of breath. She looks much older than her age and she is very frail. She is tachypnoeic and there is widespread wheez on auscultation. Blood results show raised inflammatory markers and ABG on air shows:

- PO_2 5.9 kPa
- PCO_2 7.1 kPa
- H^+ 43 nmol/L
- HCO_3^- 38 mmol/L

01. What do the ABG results show?

02. Name 4 chest X-ray abnormalities you would expect to see.

COMPLETE CDM KEY

03. What is your immediate management?

COMPLETE CDM KEY

RESPIRATORY

CASE 3
SCENARIO

A 21-year-old man with a history of asthma presents with 3 days of increasing shortness of breath and wheeze. He is distressed and unable to complete sentences when trying to answer your questions. Auscultation reveals reduced air entry throughout. His observations are:

- HR (bpm) 135
- BP (mmHg) 95/50
- RR 32.

01. You are the on-call medical FY1. What is your immediate management plan?

RESPIRATORY

CASE 4

SCENARIO

A 32-year-old man experience sharp left chest pain with associated shortness of breath. On examination he is distressed and breathless. The trachea is central, but he is hyper-resonant on percussion on the left side.

01. What is your Initial diagnosis?

02. What is your immediate management plan?

COMPLETE CDM KEY

RESPIRATORY

CASE 5

SCENARIO

COMPLETE CDM KEY

You are the on-call medical FY2. You are paged by A&E to review a 75-year-old man who has presented with increasing shortness of breath. From his examination, the A%E FY2 thinks the patient might have a pleural effusion.

01. As you walk to A&E, you try recall the clinical signs of pleural effusion. Can you give 4 signs that may be present?

    _____

    _____

    _____

    _____

02. What 2 investigation would you perform to confirm the diagnosis?

    _____

    _____

03. Effusions are either transudate or exudate. What does this mean?

    _____

    _____

04. Give 6 causes of a pleural effusion and list if transudate or exudate.

05. If examination of the pleural fluid does not confirm diagnosis, what further investigation could be consideration?

Your patient initially improves and is discharged. However, he is unfortunately readmitted with a recurrence of the effusion.

06. What further measures can be taken to reduce the frequency of the fluid collecting again in the future?

COMPLETE CDM KEY

# COMPLETE CDM KEY

RESPIRATORY

CASE 6

SCENARIO

A 19-year-old man presents to A&E with an 8-hour history of increasing shortness of breath, haemoptysis and left-sided pleuritic chest pain. He flew back from New Zealand yesterday. He looks unwell and cyanosed. His respiratory rate is 30 and heart rate is 120. He is apyrexial and has a BP of 100/50 mmHg.

01. What are your top 2 differential diagnoses?

02. What urgent investigation would you request?

COMPLETE CDM KEY

03. Give 2 likely precipitating causes for your differentials from question 1.

03. For the most likely diagnosis, give 2 immediate therapies which would be appropriate.

COMPLETE CDM KEY

RESPIRATORY

CASE 7

SCENARIO

A 22-years-old man with a history of asthma is admitted with a 4-hour history of increasing shortness of breath and wheeze. He looks distressed and you decide to do an ABG (reference ranges in brackets):

- PaO_2 8.4kPa (10.5-14kPa)
- $PaCO_2$ 4.1kPa (4.7-6kPa)
- pH.   7.53 (7.37-7.42)
- H^+ 33nmol/L (35-45nmol/L)
- HCO_3^- 25mmol/L (24-28mmol/L)
-

01. You continue your history and examination. What 6 features will assist you in assessing the severity of the asthma attack?

02. What 3 immediate therapeutic interventions would you commence?

COMPLETE CDM KEY

03. Explain the ABG results to a medical student who is attached to your ward.

04. The patient doesn't respond to your initial management plan. You repeat an ABG. What would you expect it to show?

COMPLETE CDM KEY

03. Your patient continues to deteriorate despite your best efforts. What will you do?

_____

_____

_____

_____

RESPIRATORY

CASE 8

SCENARIO

A 69-years-old man has had a total knee replacement. He completes physio and is discharged. His only new medication a tramadol. Five days later he presents to A&E with left-sided pleuritic chest pain. He has a productive cough with yellow, blood-streaked sputum.

01. What are your top 2 differential diagnoses?

02. You carry out an ECG. The registrar thinks it's consistent with pulmonary embolus. She puts you on the spot and asks you to name three features from the ECG that would be in keeping with PE – which do you suggest?

COMPLETE CDM KEY

03. Name 2 quick investigations which would help to confirm the diagnosis.

04. The patient looks breathless and sore, so you administer oxygen and analgesia. What further treatment should the patient receive?

05. After a lengthy discussion, the consultant discharges the patient on warfarin. What advice would you give your patient regarding their warfarin therapy?

COMPLETE CDM KEY

RESPIRATORY

CASE 9

SCENARIO

A 56-years-old man who is a heavy smoker presents with cough, weight loss and haemoptysis. You are concerned that his symptoms may be secondary to lung cancer.

01. What two radiological investigations would you arrange?

02. Histology is needed for confirmation. How is this obtained?

03. Name 2 other reasons for obtaining histology.

04. Give 4 histological types of lung cancer.

05. Name a specific lung tumour type that is particularly chemo-responsive?

All the multi-disciplinary team (MDT) meeting, the decision is made to operate on the tumour.

05. Give 4 factors that would classify a tumour as operable.

COMPLETE CDM KEY

RESPIRATORY

CASE 10

SCENARIO

You are called to A&E to assess a 70-year-old man. He has a history of lung cancer that was resected 2 year ago. He presents with a 3-week history of back pain that has been progressively getting worse. He has been referred today by his GP because he is now complaining of weakness and numbness in his legs. The GP has referred to hospital to exclude spinal metastases and cord compression.

01. What other functional disturbance would you expect to find?

02. Examination reveals features in keeping with an upper motor neuron lesion. Give 4 features that would support this.

03. You organize an urgent MRI which confirms spinal cord compression. This is a palliative care emergency. What 3 therapeutic interventions should be considered?

COMPLETE CDM KEY

04. The patient is admitted to the word when you receive a phone call from biochemistry. The patient's calcium is markedly raised. Give two possible reasons for this.

05. Name 2 histological types of lung cancer. (2 Marks)

COMPLETE CDM KEY

RESPIRATORY

CASE 11

SCENARIO

A 77-year-old lady and heavy smoker presents with increasing shortness of breath, haemoptysis and weight loss. Initial bloods reveal a sodium of 112mmol/L.

01. Give 2 early symptoms of hyponatraemia.

02. Give 2 effects that severe hyponatraemia can cause.

03. Name 4 common causes of hyponatraemia.

COMPLETE CDM KEY

04. What is the most likely cause of hyponatraemia in this patient?

05. Outline the immediate management of hyponatraemia.

06. Give 3 relevant investigations in this case and say what findings you would expect for each of these.

COMPLETE CDM KEY

RESPIRATORY

ANSWERS

Case 1: COPD

01. **COPD is a disease of:**
    - Emphysema
    - Chronic bronchitis

02. **Pathophysiology of COPD:**
    - **Chronic bronchitis:**
        - Goblet cell hyperplasia and mucous gland hypertrophy, leading to mucus hypersecretion.
        - Smooth muscle hypertrophy and chronic airway inflammation leads to airway fibrosis and remodeling with loss of cilia and squamous metaplasia.
    - **Emphysema:**
        - Dilation of airspaces distal to terminal bronchioles with destruction of alveolar walls
        - Air trapping due to loss of elastic recoil of lung and collapse of small airways

03. **Investigations in COPD:**
    - **Spirometry:** FEV_1 <80% predicted and FEV_1/FVC <70% with <u>little or no reversibility</u>
    - **Chest X-ray:** hyperinflation (>6 interior ribs above diaphragm in mid-clavicular line); flattened diaphragms; decreased peripheral vascular marking with distended pulmonary arteries; bullae
    - **ABG:** reduced $PaO_2 \pm$ hypercapnia – usually a type II respiratory failure.

COMPLETE CDM KEY

04. **Smoking cessation:**

    - Nicotine gum
    - Transdermal nicotine patches
    - Varenicline: oral selective nicotine receptor partial agonist
    - Bupropion (increases quit rate to 30% at 1 year)
    - Support groups (and other smoking cessation services, e.g. national helplines, pharmacy services)
    - Motivational interviewing-brief intervention

05. **Inhalers in COPD:**

    - Ventolin (salbutamol): B_2 agonist which enhances the action of noradrenaline on bronchial B-receptors causing smooth muscle relaxation
    - Spiriva (tiotroplum bromide) / Atrovent (ipratroplum bromid) antimuscarinics which inhibit parasympathetic-mediated bronchoconstrictio

Case 2: COPD

01. **ABG results show:**

    - Type 2 respiratory failure with compensatory metabolic alkalosis

02. **CXR findings in COPD:**

    - Lung hyperinflation (>6 anterior ribs seen above diaphragm in mid-clavicular line, >10 posterior ribs)
    - Flat hemidiaphragms
    - Large central pulmonary arteries with reduced peripheral vascular markings
    - Bullae

03. **Immediate management:**

    - Assess ABCDE

COMPLETE CDM KEY

- Controlled oxygen therapy: start at 24-28%; titrate according to ABGs –aim for sats of 88-92% (monitor O_2 sats and ABGs)
- Nebulised bronchodilator with oxygen: salbutamol (5mg) and ipratropium bromide (0.5mg)
- Gain IV access and take FBC, U&Es, CRP, blood and sputum cultures
- IV hydrocortisone 200mg
- Antibiotics (as per local guidelines-IV amoxicillin and oral clarithromycin)
- Arrange CXR and ECG
- If not improving, call senior / ITU for help and consider repeating nebulisers, IV aminophylline, NIV, intubation and ventilation

COMPLETE CDM KEY

Case 3: Acute asthma

01. **Management of acute asthma**
    - Assess ABCDE and **call for senior help!**
    - Ensure monitoring of HR, BP, RR, oxygen saturation and PEFR if possible.
    - Sit patient up and start high flow oxygen: 100% via non-rebreathing mask.
    - Give nebulised salbutamol 5mg and ipratropium bromide 0.5mg with oxygen
    - Gain IV access: take bloods (FBC, U&Es, CRP) and give IV hydrocortisone 200mg
    - Do an ABG; arrange chest X-ray and ECG
    - Repeat nebulisers as necessary every 15 mins ('back-to-back')
    - Consider IV magnesium sulphate and aminophylline loading does (if not on oral theophylline), or IV salbutamol if condition is not improving – after discussion with senior
    - Inform ITU for consideration of intubation and ventilation

COMPLETE CDM KEY

Case 4: Left-sided pneumothorax

01. **Likely diagnosis:** left sided pneumothorax

02. **Immediate management of pneumothorax:**
    - ABCDE approach and monitor HR, RR, O_2 sats
    - Give 100% oxygen via trauma mask
    - Gain IV access take bloods (FBC, U&Es, CRP)
    - Arrange investigations: ABG; ECG
    - PA chest X-ray to confirm pneumothorax
    - If confirmed not to be tension pneumothorax: aspirate, then monitor for recurrence
    - If unsuccessful repeat aspiration if <2.5L was aspirated on first attempt, or insert chest drain in 5th intercostal space, mid-axillary line above the rib below, with a 14F chest drain using a sterile Seldinger technique
    - Attach drain below level of chest with free end inserted into underwater one-way valve (watch for bubbling / swinging on cough: indicates air moving); should stay in place until lung re-expands and drain has stopped bubbling for 24h
    - Followed by chest X-ray and follow-up in respiratory clinic at 7-10 days: cannot fly for 6 weeks, and avoid diving

Case 5: Pleural effusion

01. **Clinical signs of pleural effusion:**

    - Reduced chest expansion on side of effusion
    - Stony dull percussion over area of effusion
    - Diminished breath sounds over area of effusion
    - Decreased vocal resonance and tactile vocal fremitus

02. **Investigations in pleural effusion:**

    - Chest X-ray
    - Ultrasound-guided diagnostic aspiration of fluid

03. **Transudate vs. exudate:**

    - Transudate: an effusion containing <25g/L of protein
    - Exudate: contains >35mg/L of protein
    - If protein levels are between these values then look at the pleural fluid protein : serum protein ratio; if >0.5 then it's and exudate

04. **Causes of pleural effusion:**

    - **Transudates:**
        - Increased venous pressure: cardiac failure (left ventricular or congestive); fluid overload; constrictive pericarditis
        - Hypoalbuminaemia: liver failure; nephrotic syndrome; malabsorption
    - **Exudates** (caused by an increase in capillary leakiness due to infection malignancy or inflammation):
        - Infection: pneumonia, TB
        - Pulmonary infarct
        - Rheumatoid arthritis / systemic lupus erythematosus
        - Malignancy : breast / bronchial carcinoma, mesothelioma, lymphoma

05. **Further investigation in pleural effusion:**

COMPLETE CDM KEY

- Pleural biopsy

06. **Reducing the frequency of pleural effusion:**

- Pleurodesis (tetracycline, bleomycin or talc)
- Long-term pleural drain in pleuroperitoneal shunt
- Pleurectomy

Case 6: Pulmonary embolism

01. **Differential: dyspnea, pleuritic chest pain and haemoptysis:**

- Pulmonary embolism
- Pneumothorax

02. **Immediate investigations:**

- Bloods: FBC, U&Es, coagulation screen, D-dimer
- ABG (type 1 respiratory failure – low PaO_2 and low/normal $paCO_2$) and oxygen saturations
- Chest X-ray
- ECG

03. **Precipitating factors**

- Pulmonary embolism: history of recent long-haul flight (venous stasis) and dehydration
- Spontaneous pneumothorax: young fit male with idiopathic sulbplerual bullae and asthma.

04. **Likely diagnosis is PE:**

- Oxygen (100% through non-rebreathing mask)
- Gain IV access and give LMWH (e.g enoxaparin 1.5mg / kg/24h SC) and start warfarin/apixaban (after diagnosis confirmed on CTPA)

Case 7: Type 2 respiratory failure

01. **Assessing asthma severity – features from history and examination:**

- Whether he can talk: in full sentences, in short phrases or not at all
- Respiratory rate: >25/min, feeble respiratory effort
- Heart rate: >110bpm, or bradycardia
- Blood pressure: hypotension
- Cyanosis
- Breath sounds: polyphonic wheeze, silent chest
- Exhaustion, confusion, or coma
- Peak expiratory flow rate: <50% (severe attack); <33% (life-threatening)

02. **Immediate therapeutic interventions in asthma:**

- Sit patient up and give high flow oxygen (15L/min) through non-rebreathing mask
- Nebulised salbutamol (5mg) and ipratroplum bromide (0.5mg) with oxygen- 'back-to-back'
- Steroids: IV hydrocortisone 200mg

03. **Explaining the initial ABG in early asthma:**

- **Low PaO$_2$**: airway constriction means less air reaches alveoli, so decreased O$_2$ exchange
- **Low PaCO$_2$**: low paO$_2$ and panic stimulates respiration, therefore hyperventilation blows off CO$_2$
- **Low H$^+$ / high pH:** H$^+$ is lost through bicarbonate buffer system thus low H$^+$ and high pH. Bicarbonate is also lost here as CO$_2$ depleted (**low HCO$_2$**)

04. **Deteriorating ABG in asthma-type 2 respiratory failure:**

- PaO$_2$ falls (hypoxia) PaCO$_2$ rises (hypercapnia) and pH will fall (acidotic)

05. **If your patient continues to deteriorate:**

COMPLETE CDM KEY

- Contact senior help and ITU for consideration of intubation and ventilation!
- IV management. Consider IV aminophylline and IV salbutamol (after discussion with a senior)

Case 8: Pulmonary embolism

01. **Differential diagnosis – post-op pleuritic chest pain and productive cough / haemoptysis:**

    - Pulmonary
    - Pneumonia

02. **ECG changes in pulmonary embolism:**

    - Right bundle branch block (RBBB)
    - Right ventricular strain pattern (right axis deviation, dominant R waves in V1 + V2, T wave inversion in V1 + V2 ST depression in V1 + V2)
    - The rare SI QIII TIII morphology (deep S waves in I, pathologic Q waves in III, inverted T waves in III)
    - Sinus tachycardia – may be only ECG finding

03. **Investigation:**

    - D-dimer
    - Chest X-ray
    - CT pulmonary angiogram (definitive diagnostic investigation in pulmonary embolism)

04. **Treatment of pulmonary embolism:** low molecular weight heparin

05. **Warfarin advice:**

    - Do not drink more than 2 units of alcohol per day
    - If you become, unwell, or start a new medication, get you INR checked
    - Never take aspirin or NSAIDs, take paracetamol instead
    - Always inform pharmacists, nurses and doctors that you are on warfarin
    - If you have a head injury with drowsiness, vomiting, headache, or nosebleed >15 mins, go to A&E

Case 9: Lung cancer

COMPLETE CDM KEY

01. **Radiological investigations:**
    - Chest X-ray
    - CT (chest, abdo, pelvis for staging)

02. **Histology is obtained via:** bronchoscopy with biopsy

03. **Histology confirms diagnosis and gives:** tumour type and grade

04. **Histological lung cancer types:**
    - Small cell
    - Large cell
    - Adenocarcinoma
    - Squamous

05. **Small cell lung cancer is chemo-responsive**

06. **Operable lung cancer:**
    - Tumour confined to lung parenchyma and over 2cm away from carina
    - Non-small cell tumour
    - No nodal involvement or distant metastases
    - Normal pulmonary function (assessed on spirometry) and no significant co-morbidity

Case 10: Lung cancer

01. **Spinal cord compression** = back pain + leg

    Weakness / paraesthesia + sphincter dysfunction: leading to incontinence (urinary ± faecal) or urinary retention

02. **Upper motor neurone lesion:**
    - Increased tone (clasp knife)
    - Clonus
    - Hyper-reflexia
    - Upgoing plantars / Babinski positive

03. **Therapeutic options in spinal cord compression:**
    - Lie patient flat and give high dose dexamethasone 8-16mg IV
    - Surgery: spinal decompression
    - Local radiotherapy

04. **Causes of hypercalcaemia in cancer:**
    - Direct invasion of tumour into bone causing release of calcium and activating osteoclasts to increase bone resorption
    - Secretion of PTHrP (PTH-related peptide) as paraneoplastic effect of tumour causing increased calcium uptake from gut and increased bone resorption

05. **Lung cancer Type:**
    - Small cell
    - Squamous cell

COMPLETE CDM KEY

Case 11: Hyponatraemia

01. **Initial symptoms of mild hyponatraemia:**
    - Nausea
    - Muscle weakness
    - Confusion

02. **Severe hyponatraemia:**
    - Seizures
    - Coma

03. **Causes of hyponatraemia:**
    - Fluid overload (either orally or as excess 5% dextrose
    - Syndrome of inappropriate ADH (SIADH)
    - Diuretics (thiazides)
    - Malignancy (small cell, prostate, pancreas, lymphoma)
    - Fluid losses: diarrhea, burns
    - Addison's disease

04. **Causes of hypercalcaemia in this case:**
    - SIADH from malignancy – paraneoplastic effect of small cell lung cancer

05. **Management of hyponatraemia:**
    - If possible, correct underlying cause
    - Check serum and urine osmolality and urinary sodium; glucose, TFTs, short synacthen test (SST), myeloma screen
    - If serum osmolality <285mmol/L then assess fluid status
    - Hypovolaemic hyponatraemia, restore volume with isotonic sodium chloride 0.9% IV

- Euvolaemic or hypervolaemic: stop relevant medications; 1.5 L/day fluid restriction ; consider IV NaCl or demeclocycline (senior decision)

06. **Investigations:**

    - Chest X-ray; may show 'coin lesion; hilar enlargement or pleural effusion
    - Bronchoscopy: lesion
    - CT: may show position of cancerous lesion and any metastases / lymph node involvement

COMPLETE CDM KEY

CHAPTER

GASTROENTEROLOGY

CASE 1

SCENARIO

A 64-year-old woman presents to A&E with severe upper abdominal pain radiating to her back. Examination reveals generalised abdominal tenderness and guarding in the epigastric region. Her amylase is 2360units/dL. You suspect acute pancreatitis.

01. What are the 2 most common causes of acute pancreatitis?

_____

_____

_____

_____

To risk stratify the patient, you work out the patient's Glasgow-lmrie score using the following results: WCC 20.0×10^9 /L, glucose 4.2

COMPLETE CDM KEY

mmol/L, LDH 370iu/L, urea 9.0mmol/L, calcium 2.2mmol/L, PaO$_2$ 7.7kPa.

02. Based on the results above your registrar asks if this is mild, moderate or severe pancreatitis – what do you think?

_____

_____

COMPLETE CDM KEY

03. What is your immediate management?

04. Your patient deteriorates despite maximal medical therapy. Give 4 life-threatening complications of acute pancreatitis.

COMPLETE CDM KEY

05. Your consultant decides that your patient needs surgery. What is an indication for surgery in a patient with server pancreatitis?

GASTROENTEROLOGY

CASE 2

SCENARIO

A 32-year-old man, who fell off his bike, presents with left upper quadrant pain radiating to his left shoulder tip. His pulse is 105bpm and his systolic BP is 89mmHg.

01. You are the FY2 assessing the patient in A&E and make a rapid assessment of ABC. Outline 4 immediate measures you would take.

02. You suspect a splenic injury. What radiological investigation do you order to confirm the diagnosis?

03. Other than splenectomy, name 2 other management options for splenic injury.

04. Name 3 diseases which predispose to splentic rupture.

Your patient undergoes splenectomy and you assist the consultant in theatre.

05. Your consultant asks you what 2 medical therapies are mandatory following splenectomies?

GASTROENTEROLOGY

CASE 3

SCENARIO

A 57-year-old man is admitted with a 5-day history of melaena and abdominal distension. On examination, appears confused, he has multiple spider naevi, hepatoplenomegaly and gross ascites. Bloods show:

- Hb — 9d/dl
- WCC — $3.2 \times 10^9/L$
- Platelets — $72 \times 10^9/L$
- Albumin — 21g/L
- Bilirubin — 14umol/L
- Alkaline phosphatase — 410iu/L
- ALT — 157iu/L

You organize an abdominal ultrasound which shows irregular liver edge, splenomegaly and ascites.

01. What is the most likely cause of the melaena?

02. What is the name given to the confusion in this case?

03. Give 3 possible precipitating factors for the acute confusion and outline appropriate treatment for each causes.

04. Give 3 Management options for treating the ascites.

05. The patient develops asterixis and so, on the ward round, the consultant asks you to name 2 other causes of assterixis.

COMPLETE CDM KEY

GASTROENTEROLOGY

CASE 4

SCENARIO

A 69-year-old woman presents with a 2-month history of epigastric pain radiating to her back. She has been losing weight and CT shows a mass at the head of the pancreas.

01. On the word round, your consultant asks you the 2 main functions of the pancreas and to give 2 examples of each function.

02. You examine the patient's gastrointestinal system-list 6 signs you might expect to find.

COMPLETE CDM KEY

03. At the MDT meeting, the team are discussing management options. What is the most likely operation for this type of tumour?

04. Sadly the tumour is inoperable, so list 3 symptomatic measures that can be taken to relieve the patient's symptoms.

GASTROENTEROLOGY

CASE 5

SCENARIO

A 57-year-old man presents to A&E with periumbilical pain radiating to the left iliac fossa. He describes a history of intermittent constipation and fresh PR bleeding. Examination reveals tenderness in the LIF.

01. What is the most likely diagnosis? Describe the disease process.

02. What are the differences between the congenital and acquired forms of this condition?

Your patient improves and is discharged after conservative measures. Two weeks later, he is readmitted with fever and abdominal pain. When you examine him, he is extremely tender in the LIF with localized guarding and rigidity. You think you can feel a mass in the LIF.

03. What is the most likely cause for his new symptoms?

COMPLETE CDM KEY

04. Bloods reveal elevated inflammatory markers. Name 2 other investigations that could help confirm your diagnosis.

05. What is your immediate medical management?

COMPLETE CDM KEY

06. Name 2 complications of the disease that would require surgical intervention.

_____

___ _____

___ _____

___ _____

COMPLETE CDM KEY

GASTROENTEROLOGY

CASE 6

SCENARIO

A 71-year-old man presents with weight loss, new constipation and PR bleeding. You are concerned that he may have colorectal cancer.

01. Name 2 other possible causes of the rectal bleeding.

02. What 4 investigations would you perform on this patient?

03. Give 4 risk factors for developing colorectal cancer.

COMPLETE CDM KEY

04. What scale is used for classification of colorectal cancer?

05. What 2 criteria does this scale use in classification?

06. Briefly outline the management of colorectal cancer.

COMPLETE CDM KEY

GASTROENTEROLOGY

CASE 7

SCENARIO

A 54-year-old woman presents with right upper quadrant pain that radiates to her back. She has a temperature of 38.1 °C. You suspect acute cholecystitis.

01. Name 3 other differential diagnoses for the patient's symptoms.

02. What investigation would confirm the diagnosis and what would you expect it to show?

COMPLETE CDM KEY

The diagnosis is confirmed.

COMPLETE CDM KEY

03. After you gain IV access. What 3 immediate therapies would you prescribe?

_____

_____

_____

_____

_____

_____

The consultant decides that the patient needs a laparoscopic cholecystectomy.

04. What are the 2 most common complications associated with this procedure?

_____

_____

_____

_____

GASTROENTEROLOGY

CASE 8

SCENARIO

A 9-year-old girl is brought to A&E with a short history of abdominal pain and fever. She is tender in the right iliac fossa with localised guarding.

01. What is the most likely diagnosis?

02. What other features from the history would support your diagnosis?

03. What other examination features would support your diagnosis?

COMPLETE CDM KEY

What you are examining the patient. She suddenly complains of increased abdominal pain. Her abdomen is rigid. The nurse repeats observations and she is tachycardic and hypotensive.

04. What is the most likely cause of her deterioration?

05. Give 2 findings on examination or investigation which would support your diagnosis.

06. You call the registrar. After assessing ABCDE, she asks you what 2 therapeutic measures should be undertaken.

COMPLETE CDM KEY

COMPLETE CDM KEY

GASTROENTEROLOGY

CASE 9

SCENARIO

You see a 52-year-old man in clinic with chronic pancreatitis and insufficiency.

01. As food enters the digestive tract, hormones are released from the stomach and duodenum. Name 3 examples of these hormones.

02. Most digestive enzymes are secreted from the pancreas as proenzymes of zymogens. Why is this advantageous?

03. Describe the anatomical route through which pancreatic secretions leave the pancreas.

04. Which constituent of pancreatic secretions mostly determines its pH?

05. Why is this constituent particularly important?

06. List 3 pancreatic substances that act to digest proteins / peptides.

COMPLETE CDM KEY

COMPLETE CDM KEY

GASTROENTEROLOGY

CASE 10

SCENARIO

A 64-year-old man presents to A&E after vomiting fresh red blood. He drinks 40 units of alcohol per week. He looks pale and clammy.

01. What 3 physiological observations will help you to determine the severity of the haematemesis?

02. What is your initial management?

03. What investigations would you carry out?

COMPLETE CDM KEY

04. Name the 2 most likely causes of the bleeding.

05. Your patient is haemodynamically unstable. What therapeutic intervention is needed to achieve haemostasis?

Bloods come back showing a coagulopathy which you attribute to his alcohol intake.

06. Name 2 parameters that are likely to be abnormal and state why.

COMPLETE CDM KEY

GASTROENTEROLOGY

CASE 11

SCENARIO

A 50-year-old man presents with a 3-month history of pain when swallowing. He says that food is getting 'stuck'. He has lot 7kg in weight. He is a lifelong smoker. He drinks 4 pints of beer every night. You think that he might have oesophageal cancer.

01. Give 4 other different diagnoses that can cause dysphagia.

02. What 2 features from a patient's history would make you think that the dysphagia is caused by malignancy?

03. You are asked to organise some investigations – which 2 would confirm the diagnosis?

COMPLETE CDM KEY

04. On the ward round, the registrar asks you to name the 2 main histological types of oesophageal carcinoma.

The patient's case is discussed at the MDT meeting. The team considers a surgical resection for this man's oesophageal carcinoma.

05. Which investigations is now important and why?

06. Unfortunately, surgical resection isn't possible, so provide 2 measures to manage the patient's symptoms.

COMPLETE CDM KEY

GASTROENTEROLOGY

CASE 12

SCENARIO

A 42-year-old man presents to his GP with a history of epigastric pain. The GP suspects he has a gastric ulcer.

01. *H. pylori* infection can predispose to gastric ulceration; give 2 other risk factors for peptic ulcer disease.

02. Describe the histological changes found in gastric ulcers.

The GP investigations for *H. pylori* infection

COMPLETE CDM KEY

03. What non-invasive test can be performed to confirm the presence of *H.pylori*?

_____

_____

H. pylori is confirmed. The GP discusses treatment with the patient.

04. What treatment regime should he commence? Give 2 specific typed of drugs.

_____

_____

_____

_____

Three months later the patient is admitted with projectile vomiting containing recently ingested food. You suspect he has developed gastric outflow obstruction.

05. What investigation would you use to confirm the diagnosis?

_____

_____

COMPLETE CDM KEY

06. What is your immediate management?

GASTROENTEROLOGY

CASE 12

SCENARIO

A 42-year-old man presents to his GP with a history of epigastric pain. The GP suspects he has a gastric ulcer.

01. *H. pylori* infection can predispose to gastric ulceration; give 2 other risk factors for peptic ulcer disease.

02. Describe the histological changes found in gastric ulcers.

The GP investigations for *H. pylori* infection

COMPLETE CDM KEY

03. What non-invasive test can be performed to confirm the presence of *H.pylori*?

_____

_____

H. pylori is confirmed. The GP discusses treatment with the patient.

04. What treatment regime should he commence? Give 2 specific typed of drugs.

_____

_____

_____

_____

Three months later the patient is admitted with projectile vomiting containing recently ingested food. You suspect he has developed gastric outflow obstruction.

05. What investigation would you use to confirm the diagnosis?

_____

_____

COMPLETE CDM KEY

06. What is your immediate management?

GASTROENTEROLOGY

CASE 13

SCENARIO

A 59-year-old woman presents with a 4-month history of epigastric pain which is exacerbated by eating.

01. Name 3 organs which may cause food-related pain.

When you examine the patient there is mild tenderness in the epigastrium, but Murphy's sign is negative.

02. Your consultant asks you to explain the significance of Murphy's sign.

COMPLETE CDM KEY

03. You want to exclude *H. Pylori*. What basic investigation would you request?

H.pylori is confirmed and you commence triple therapy.

04. Outline the pharmacological action of lansoprazole.

05. Give 2 complications of peptic ulceration.

You have just finished writing the patient's discharge summary when the nurse urgently call you to the patient's bedside. The patient looks unwell and is complaining of severe abdominal pain. Her abdomen is rigid. You suspect perforation.

COMPLETE CDM KEY

06. What investigation should be performed to support your provisional diagnosis?

GASTROENTEROLOGY

CASE 14

SCENARIO

A 24-year-old man is admitted with a 4-day history of diarrhea. He describes blood and mucus mixed in his stool. He also complains of severe cramping abdominal pain. On examination he looks unwell with dry, cracked lips. His pulse is 100bpm and his temperature is 38.2 °C.

01. What is your immediate management plan?

02. Give 3 investigations you would order.

COMPLETE CDM KEY

03. You think he may have ulcerative colitis – which 2 medical treatments would you institute immediately?

    _____

    ____

    _____

    ____

    _____

    _____

    ____

04. Name 2 major complications of ulcerative colitis.

    _____

    ____

    _____

    ____

05. Your consultant thinks he might need an operation – which 2 surgical procedures might be indicated?

    _____

    ____

    _____

    ____

    _____

COMPLETE CDM KEY

GASTROENTEROLOGY

CASE 15

SCENARIO

A 23-year-old medical student returned from an elective in India. Four days later she presents with diarrhoea. She complains of profuse, watery diarrhoea and she has noticed some blood in her stools. She pyrexial and there is generalised abdominal tenderness. You take bloods which show haemoglobin 13.8g/dl, WCC 13×10^9/L, platelets 520×10^9/L. Kidney function is normal. CRP is 210mg/L.

01. Give 4 possible causes for her symptoms.

02. You have taken bloods for FBC, U&E, CRP, ESR. Give 3 other investigations that you would request.

COMPLETE CDM KEY

03. List 3 complications associated with dysentery.

04. Give 2 treatments for diarrhoea caused by Clostridium difficile.

COMPLETE CDM KEY

GASTROENTEROLOGY

CASE 16

SCENARIO

A 73-year-old woman attends her GP with a 4-month history of loose stools and PR bleeding. Rectal examination reveals a hard lesion in the rectum. The patient is referred for a colonoscopy and biopsies confirm rectal adenocarcinoma.

You organise a CT chest, abdomen and pelvis which shows no evidence of metastases. The patient had bowel preparation with sodium picosulfate (Picolax). Whilst you insert a cannula, the patient discusses the experience in details.

01. Name 2 common biochemical abnormalities that can occur following bowel preparation.
    _____
    _____
    _____
    _____

The consultant discusses management on the ward round. He is planning an anterior resection possibly with loop ileostomy.

02. He asks you to point out where the typical site for an ileostomy is?
    _____

COMPLETE CDM KEY

03. Give 2 features on the abdominal wall that should be avoided when siting an ileostomy.

The patient has an anterior resection. Three days later, she complains of increasing abdominal pain. She looks unwell and is tachypnoeic and pyrexial.

04. What operative complication do you need to consider?

You order a chest X-ray which shows that she has a post-op chest infection.

05. Name 2 key aspects of treatment.

COMPLETE CDM KEY

Histology of the resected bowel shows a T3, N1, R0 tumour.

06. What Dukes' stage does this equate to and what does the R0 classification mean?

07. What other therapy is likely to be advised for this patient?

GASTROENTEROLOGY

CASE 17

SCENARIO

A 65-year-old man presents with an 8-week history of lethargy. He has lost almost a stone in weight. He denies any change in bowel habit, but he has noticed pale stools. He smokes 15 cigarettes per day and drinks 8 pints of beer per week.

Blood results show:

- Bilirubin   89umol/L
- Albumin   32g/L
- AST   76iu/L
- ALT   166iu/L
- Alkaline phosphatase 346iu/L
- Hb   13.1g/dl
- WCC   6.7x 10^9/L
- Platelets   254x10^9/L
- Na   139mmol/L
- K   4.0mmol/L
- Urea   9.4mmol/L
- Creatinine   198mmol/L

01. On further examination, the patient looks jaundiced – what type of jaundice does he have? Explain how you arrived at your answer.

02. What are your top 3 differential diagnoses?

The FY2 in A&E organised an abdominal X-ray that doesn't show any specific abnormalities.

03. What 3 other investigations would you request?

COMPLETE CDM KEY

The patient is admitted and, unfortunately, endoscopic brush cytology shows the presence of malignant cells. The MDT considers surgery.

04. List 3 complications of surgery, which would be <u>specifically</u> associated with the patient's altered liver function.

___

CT shows a mass measuring 3 x 4 x 2.5cm in the pancreatic head.

05. If the patient was to undergo surgery, name 3 specific precautions or investigations that would be undertaken in view of his altered liver function.

COMPLETE CDM KEY

Further investigations shows that the mass surrounds major vessels and there are lesions in the live. The consultant decides that surgery is inappropriate. The patient's wife asks to speak to you. She wants to know the diagnosis in full and asks why her husband can't have surgery. She seems angry and is understandably upset. She demands to know why the diagnosis was not established earlier.

06. What is the most likely diagnosis?

07. Give 3 reasons why surgical resection is inappropriate.

COMPLETE CDM KEY

08. Why was the diagnosis not established earlier?

COMPLETE CDM KEY

GASTROENTEROLOGY

ANSWERS

Case 1: Acute pancreatitis

01. **Most common cause of pancreatitis in the Western world:**
    - Gallstones (-35%)
    - Ethanol (-35%)

02. **Glasgow-Imrie score:** severe

    If **three or more** of the following factors are present within the first 48 hours of onset, this suggests severe pancreatitis:

    - $\underline{P}aO_2$ <8kPa
    - $\underline{A}$ge > 55years
    - $\underline{N}$eutrophils – WCC>15x10^9/L
    - $\underline{C}$alcium <2mmol/L
    - $\underline{R}$enal function – urea > 16 mmol/L
    - $\underline{E}$nzymes – LDH >600iu/L; AST >200iu/L
    - $\underline{A}$lbumin <32g/L (serum)
    - $\underline{S}$ugar – serum glucose > 10mmol/L

03. **Immediate management of acute pancreatitis:**
    - Make patient nil by mouth and consider inserting an NG tube (reduce pancreatic stimulation)
    - Gain IV access and give IV fluid (e.g. 0.9% saline) to replace third space losses; insert urinary catheter
    - Analgesia and anti-emetic- IV morphine and IV cyclizine
    - Monitor: HR, BP, urine output, FBC, U&Es, Ca^{2+}, glucose, amylase, ABG

- If worsening, contact ITU – may require inotropes / organ support

04. **Complication of acute pancreatitis:**
    - Hypovolaemic shock
    - Renal failure
    - Sepsis: may also lead to disseminated intravascular coagulation (DIC)
    - Audit respiratory distress syndrome (ARDS)
    - Hypocalcaemia

05. **Indications for surgery:** infected pancreatic narcosis / recurrent oedematous pancreatitis.

Case 2: Ruptured spleen

01. **Immediate trauma management:**
    - Give 100% oxygen via trauma mask and make patient nil by mouth
    - Gain wide-bore IV access (x2): take blood for FBC, U&Es, LFTs, glucose, cross-match/group and save
    - Consider activating major haemorrhage protocol
    - Analgesia: morphine 5-10mg IV
    - Call senior help (trauma team depending on hospital policy)

02. **Radiological investigation to confirm splenic injury:** abdominal CT

03. **Management of splenic injury:**
    - Conservative: blood / fluid replacement and regular monitoring of FBC and imaging (if a haematoma forms then may need to be removed surgically)

COMPLETE CDM KEY

- Surgical: splenic artery embolization and splenorrhaphy (splenic salvage)

04. **Diseases predisposing to splenic rupture:**
    - Sickle cell disease
    - Infectious mononucleosis
    - Malaria
    - Leukaemia

05. **Post – splenectomy measures:**
    - Long-term prophylactic antibiotics (penicillin V)
    - Update vaccination status: Hib and men C, annual influenza vaccine, pneumococcal vaccine

Case 3: Alcoholic liver disease

01. **Most likely cause of melaena in alcoholic liver disease (ALD):**
    - Bleeding varices (oesophageal or gastric)
    - Haemorrhage from peptic ulcer

02. **Confusion in ALD:** hepatic encephalopathy

03. **Precipitating causes in hepatic encephalopathy:**
    - GI haemorrhage:
        - Management: IV fluids, vitamin K, platelets, FFP and blood; arrange urgent endoscopy
    - Infection:
        - Management: treat with antibiotics; include metronidazole, neomycin or vancomycin to decrease the concentration of ammonia forming colonic bacteria

- Constipation:
  - Management: lactulose or bowel enemas to empty bowels and reduce the nitrogen load on the gut; large doses required

Other precipitating causes:

- Renal failure
- Electrolyte imbalance
- Diuretics
- Sedative drugs (benzodiazepines, antidepressants, antipsychotics)
- High dietary protein

04. **Management of ascites:**

    - Fluid restriction (1.5L/day) and salt restriction
    - Diuretics, e.g. spironolactone (add furosemide if poor response)
    - Paracentesis

05. **Causes of asterixis:**

    - Carbon dioxide retention
    - Renal failure
    - Drug related (e.g. phenytoin)

Case 4: Pancreatic tumour

01. **Pancreatic function:**

    - Exocrine gland: acini produce digestive enzymes to break down chime to allow absorption of nutrients in the small intestine
      - Trypsin breaks down proteins into smaller peptides
      - Amylase breaks down starch in oligosaccharides and secretes HCO_3 to neutralize acid chyme
    - Endocrine gland:

- Secretes insulin from β-cells of islets of Langerhans which promotes uptake of glucose into cells
- Secretes glucagon from a –cells which promotes glycogenolysis and gluconeogenesis

02. **Possible signs in pancreatic cancer:**

- Jaundice (pale stools, dark urine – obstructive)
- Palpable / enlarged gall bladder (Courvoisier's sign)
- Epigastric mass
- Hepatomegaly (metastases)
- Splenomegaly
- Lymphadenopathy
- Ascites
- Signs of alcoholic liver disease, e.g. spider naevi
- Other rarer signs: sister Mary Joseph's nodule, thrombophlebitis migrans (Trousseau's sign)

03. **Pancreatic cancer operation;** pancreatoduodenectomy (Whipple's procedure)

04. **Symptomatic management of pancreatic cancer:**

- Relief of jaundice: ERCP stenting
- Relief of duodenal obstruction; surgical gastric bypass (gastrojejunostomy)
- Analgesia: high does opiates, may need involvement from anaesthetists, e.g. for coeliac plexus blocks
- Palliative chemotherapy and /or radiotherapy
- Chlorphenamine (an antihistamine) for pruritus

Case 5: Diverticulitis

01. **Diverticular disease:** herniations of colonic mucosa have become blocked, inflamed and prone to bleeding

02. **Congenital vs. acquired:**
    - Congenital: a 'true' diverticulum consisting of an outpouching of the whole colonic wall involving the mucosa, submucosa and muscularis
    - Acquired: consists of 'false' diverticula in which only the mucosa out-pouches between weak areas in the wall of the colon

03. **Abdominal pain + fever in patient with known diverticular disease =** acute diverticulitis

04. **Investigations:**
    - Abdominal X-ray
    - CT abdomen

05. **Immediate management of acute diverticulitis:**
    - Nil by mouth
    - IV fluids
    - Analgesia
    - Antibiotics (IV amoxicillin, metronidazole and gentamicin – depends on local guidelines)

06. **Complication of diverticulitis:**
    - Perforation
    - Diverticular fistula

Case 6: Colorectal cancer

01. Causes of rectal bleeding:
- Diverticulitis
- Colorectal polyp
- Inflammatory bowel disease
- Angiodysplasia
- Ischaemic colitis
- Infective colitis

02. Investigations:
- Bloods: FBC, coagulation, LFTs, ESR/CRP, U&Es carcinoembryonic antigen (CEA)
- Colonoscopy / flexible sigmoidoscopy
- Barium enema
- Contrast – enhanced CT chest, abdomen and pelvis

03. Predisposing factors in colorectal cancer:
- Known colonic polyps / polyposis syndromes / neoplastic polyps
- Positive family history (especially APC and HNPCC genes)
- Inflammatory bowel disease: ulcerative colitis and Crohn's disease
- Increasing age
- Low fiber diet

04. Classification of colorectal cancer: Duke's classification / TNM classification

05. Criteria:
- Extent of tumour invasion of colonic wall
- Presence of metastases (lymph nodes and distant)

06. Management of colorectal cancer:
- Depends on personal factors, stage of disease, and will involve a multidisciplinary approach

- Surgery: aims to cure – surgical resection of tumour
- Radiotherapy: used pre-operatively in rectal cancer to reduce local recurrence
- Chemotherapy: adjunct to surgery if Dukes' classification stage C
- Palliative therapy: chemotherapy, radiotherapy, analgesia, anti-emetics, anti-secretory drugs, laxatives, psychosocial and spiritual support.

Case 7: Acute cholecystitis

01. **Differential diagnosis of acute cholecystitis:**

    - Other biliary disease, e.g. ascending cholangitis, biliary colic
    - Acute pancreatitis
    - Perforated duodenal ulcer

02. **Radiological investigation:**

    - Abdominal ultrasound:
        - Gall bladder wall thickening (shrunken gall bladder)
        - Pericholecystic fluid
        - Gallstones
        - Dilated common bile duct
        - Positive sonographic Murphy's sign

03. **Immediate managements:**

    - IV fluids
    - Analgesia: IV morphine plus anti-emetic therapy
    - Antibiotics

04. **Complications of laparoscopic cholecystectomy:**

    - Conversion to open operation
    - Bile duct injury

Case 8: Acute appendicitis

01. **RIF pain and fever in paediatric** = acute appendicitis

02. **Appendicitis features:**
    - Abdominal pain: initially central, then radiating to right iliac fossa; worse on movement and coughing
    - Anorexia
    - Nausea and vomiting

03. **Examination findings:**
    - Guarding at McBurney's point
    - Foul smelling breath/fetor
    - Rovsing's sign: palpation in left iliac fossa causes pain in the right iliac fossa

04. **Acute deterioration in appendicitis:** perforation of appendix leading to peritonitis

05. **Clinical features of perforation:**
    - Examination:
        - Board-like rigidity across entire abdomen
        - Abdominal distension
    - Investigation:
        - Raised WCC
        - Erect chest X-ray: may show air under diaphragm

06. **Management:**
    - IV antibiotics and IV fluid resuscitation
    - Appendectomy

COMPLETE CDM KEY

Case 9: Chronic pancreatitis

01. **Digestive hormones:**

    - Gastrin (G cells, antrum of stomach)
    - CCK/cholecystokinin (duodenum)
    - Secretin (duodenum)
    - Motilin (jejunum and duodenum)
    - Gastric inhibitory polypeptide (jejunum and duodenum)
    - Somatostain from D cells (some in gastric mucosa, although mostly in endocrine pancreas)

02. **Zymogens / proenzymes:** enzymes are not activated until they reach the brush border of the duodenum, therefore this **prevents autodigestion / autolysis / self-digestion** while in the pancreas

03. **Anatomical route of pancreatic secretions:** produced in acinue of lobule → acinar duct → intercalated duct → interlobular duct → **pancreatic duct** →joins the **common bile duct** at the **ampulla of Vater** → lumen of the duodenum

04. **Pancreatic pH determined by:** bicarbonate ions (alkaline)

05. **Bicarbonate is important because it:** neutralises the gastric acid as it enters the duodenum, thus preventing duodenal irritation and ulceration

06. **Pancreatic protein digestion:**

    - Trypsin
    - Chymotrypsin
    - Elastase
    - Carboxypeptidase

COMPLETE CDM KEY

Case 10: Chronic pancreatitis

01. **Digestive hormones:**

    - Gastrin (G cells, antrum of stomach)
    - CCK/cholecystokinin (duodenum)
    - Secretin (duodenum)
    - Motilin (jejunum and duodenum)
    - Gastric inhibitory polypeptide (jejunum and duodenum)
    - Somatostain from D cells (some in gastric mucosa, although mostly in endocrine pancreas)

02. **Zymogens / proenzymes:** enzymes are not activated until they reach the brush border of the duodenum, therefore this **prevents autodigestion / autolysis / self-digestion** while in the pancreas

03. **Anatomical route of pancreatic secretions:** produced in acinue of lobule → acinar duct → intercalated duct → interlobular duct → **pancreatic duct** →joins the **common bile duct** at the **ampulla of Vater** → lumen of the duodenum

04. **Pancreatic pH determined by:** bicarbonate ions (alkaline)

05. **Bicarbonate is important because it:** neutralises the gastric acid as it enters the duodenum, thus preventing duodenal irritation and ulceration

06. **Pancreatic protein digestion:**

    - Trypsin
    - Chymotrypsin
    - Elastase
    - Carboxypeptidase

COMPLETE CDM KEY

Case 11: Alcoholic liver disease

01. **Physiological observations to assess shock:**
    - Pulse
    - Blood pressure
    - Urine output

02. **Immediate management:**
    - ABCDE and call senior help!
    - IV access with 2 wide-bore cannulas and give fluids / blood products

03. **Investigations:**
    - Bloods: FBC, U&Es, LFTs, coagulation screen, cross-match, glucose
    - ABG
    - Chest X-ray: exclude perforation

04. **Most likely causes of beleeding:**
    - Varices (oesophageal or gastric)
    - Perforated peptic ulcer

05. **oesophagogastroduodenoscopy (OGD) for haemostasis in GI bleed:** endoscopy (for haemostasis with adrenaline injection, sclerotherapy / banding depending on aetiology)

06. **Coagulopathy in ALD:**
    - Prolonged PT and APTT: due to reduced synthesis of vitamin K and clotting factors necessary for haemostasis due to liver damage
    - Platelet count (thrombocytopenia): decreased formation of platelets due to toxic effect of alcohol on platelet production and hypersplenism from portal hypertension

Case 12: Dysphagia

01. **Differential of dysphagia:**
    - Stricture
    - Tonsillitis / tonsillar abscess
    - Neurological disorder, e.g. pseudobulbar palsy, motor neurone disease, multiple sclerosis. Parkinson's disease, stroke, vagus or glossopharyngeal never injury
    - Extrinsic pressure, e.g. retrosternal goitre, lung cancer
    - Achalasia
    - Diffuse oesophageal spasm
    - Oesophageal web
    - Pharyngeal pouch
    - Foreign body

02. **Features of dysphagia that suggest malignancy:**
    - Progressive dysphagia (solids then liquids)
    - Constitutional symptoms: weight loss, anorexia, night sweats, fever
    - Known Barrett's oesophagus
    - Family history of oesophageal cancer
    - Smoker

03. **Investigations:**
    - Barium swallow ± video fluoroscopy
    - Endoscopy and biopsy

04. **Histological types:**
    - Squamous cell carcinoma
    - Adenocarcinoma

05. **Staging:** CT scan (head and neck / chest / abdo / pelvis) for staging with TNM classification: extent of tumour involvement, lymph nodes and metastases

06. **Palliative measures:**

COMPLETE CDM KEY

- Oesophageal stenting
- Chemo-radiotherapy

Case 13: Peptic ulcer disease

01. **predisposing factors in gastric ulcer:**
    - Smoking
    - Use of NSAIDs / steroids

02. **Histological changes in gastric ulceration:**
    - Layer of exudate: inflammatory cell infiltration
    - Layer of necrotic tissue with parietal cell loss
    - Layer of granulation tissue
    - Layer of dense fibrous tissue replacing muscularis propria

03. **Non-invasive investigation for H. pylori:**
    - Stool culture
    - ^{13}C-urea breath test
    - Endoscopy and biopsy

04. **Medical Management:** triple therapy with 2 antibiotics (e.g. amoxicillin / metronidazole and clarithromycin) and a proton pump inhibitor (e.g. omeprazole)

05. **Direct visualisation:** endoscopy (OGD)

06. **Management of gastric outflow obstruction:**
    - ABCDE
    - Gain IV access and give IV fluids
    - Basic investigations: FBC, U&Es, LFTs, ABG
    - Pass NG tube and aspirate stomach; make patient nil by mouth

- Proton pump inhibitor, e.g. omeprazole

Case 14: Gastric ulceration

01. **Food-related pain may arise in:**
    - Oesophagus
    - Stomach
    - Pancreas
    - Gall bladder

02. **Murphy's sign:** is indicative of inflammation of the gall bladder, i.e. acute cholecystitis

03. **Non-invasive investigation of H.pylori:** stool culture

04. **PPI mechanism of action:**
    - Lansoprazole is a proton pump inhibitor which binds to the H^+/K^+- ATPase pumps on the luminal surface of gastric parietal cells and inhibits their action
    - This prevents their normal action of secreting H^+ ions and therefore lowers the amount of acid secreted into the stomach

05. **Complication of gastric ulceration:**
    - Haemorrhage
    - Perforation
    - Stricture leading to gastric outflow obstruction
    - Malignancy

06. **Bedside investigation of perforation:** erect chest X-ray to look for air under the diaphragm

Case 15: Acute ulcerative colitis

01. **Immediate management:**
    - Make patient nil by mouth

- Gain IV access and give IV fluids: 500ml fluids challenge of 0.9 % saline followed by maintenance and replacement fluids based on vital signs with K' replacement based on U&Es
- Analgesia and anti-pyretic, e.g. paracetamol
- Regular monitoring of vital signs

02. **Investigations:**

    - Bloods: FBC, U&Es ESR/CRP, LFT, blood cultures
    - Stool microscopy, culture and sensitivity (MC&S)
    - Abdominal X-ray ± erect chest X-ray
    - Golonoscopy ± biopsy

03. **Management of acute ulcerative colitis:**

    - Steroids, e.g IV hydrocortisone 100mg/6h and rectal steroids
    - 5-ASAs: aminosalicylates, e.g. mesalazine, sulfasalazine
    - Consider immunosuppressants (e.g. infliximab) – after the acute phase

04. **Complications:**

    - Toxic megacolon which may lead to sepsis
    - Perforation and peritonitis
    - Haemorrhage
    - Increased risk of colorectal cancer
    - Venous thrombosis – hypercoagulable state

05. **Surgical options:**

    - Colectomy with loop ileostomy (can later form ileoanal pouch)
    - Proctocolectomy with end ileostomy

Case 16: Diarrhoea

01. **Bloody diarrhoea:**

    - Shigella
    - Campylobacter

- Escherichia coli
- Clostridium difficile

02. **Investigations:**

- Stool microscopy (including for ova and parasites), culture and sensitivity
- Clostridium difficile toxin
- Sigmoidoscopy / colonoscopy ($\pm$ biopsy)
- Blood cultures
- Abdominal X-ray

03. **Complications:**

- Dehydration (may lead to hypovolaemic shock)
- Electrolyte disturbance (hyponatraemia, hypokalaemia, acidosis)
- Toxic megacolon (which may lead to perforation and peritonitis)
- Sepsis
- Hepatic / brain abscess

04. **Management of C. difficile:**

- ABCDE assessment with IV fluid resuscitation and electrolyte replacement
- Antibiotics:
    - Stop pre-existing antibiotics (especially cephalosporins)
    - Start metronidazole or vancomycin

COMPLETE CDM KEY

Case 17: Rectal adenocarcinoma

01. **Biochemical abnormalities following bowel prep:**
    - Hypokalaemia
    - Hyponatraemia

02. **Ileostomy site:** right iliac fossa

03. **Abdominal features to avoid in ileostomy planning:**
    - Any previous scars
    - Skin folds / crease
    - Area of waistband
    - Umbilicus

04. **if patient deteriorates after anterior resection, always consider:** anastomotic breakdown and leakage (leading to faecal peritonitis)

05. **Managing post-op chest infection:**
    - Oxygen therapy (aim for sats>92% if no co-existing COPD)
    - Antibiotics (based on local guidelines)
    - Analgesia and chest physiotherapy

06. **Dukes' classification staging:**
    - Duke's stage C
    - R0 means that the tumour has been resected and there is no residual tumour left in the bowel (residual tumour classification)

07. **Adjuvant chemotherapy:** improves disease-free survival and overall survival in Dukes' stage C cancer

Case 18: Cholestatic jaundice

01. **Type of jaundice:**

    - Obstructive jaundice
    - Pale stools (steatorrhoea) suggests the stercobilingoen is not entering the bowel due to blockage of bile flow
    - The levels of alkaline phosphatase (an enzyme produced by biliary canaliculi) are high which is typical of any obstructive type of jaundice

02. **Causes of obstructive / cholestatic jaundice:**

    - Carcinoma in the head of the pancreas
    - Cholangiocarcinoma
    - Gallstone impacted in the common bile duct, i.e. choledocholithiasis
    - Lymph node enlargement at the porta hepatis, e.g. lymphatic spread of an abdominal malignancy
    - Cholestatic drugs, e.g. flucloxacillin, fusidic acid, chlorpromazine
    - Mirizzi syndrome-common hepatic duct obstruction cause by extrinsic compression from an impacted stone in the cystic duct or infundibulum of the gall bladder

03. **Investigations:**

    - Ultrasound of biliary tree
    - Magnetic reaonance cholangiopancreatography (MRCP) / endoscopic retrograde cholangiopancreatography (ERCP)
    - CT abdomen and pelvis
    - Coagulation screen

04. **Surgical considerations with deranged LFTs:**

    - Haemorrhage (due to coagulopathy)
    - Abnormal pharmacodynamics leading to increased risk of anaesthetic complication
    - Poor wound healing / infection (reduced production of acute phase proteins and immunoglobulins involved in the acute phase response)
    - Renal failure from hepatorenal syndrome

05. **Pre-op considerations:**

- Bloods; coagulation screen (PT, APTT), FBC (thrombocytopenia more likely)
- Broad-spectrum antibiotic prophylaxis
- Parenteral vitamin K ± fresh frozen plasma
- Careful fluid expansion pre-operatively and post-operative balance with careful calculation of drug dosages and monitoring of responses
- Pre-operative biliary decompression improves post-operative morbidity

06. **Diagnosis:** cancer of the head of the pancreas with liver metastasis

07. **Reasons why surgery may be inappropriate:**
    - Metastatic disease (i.e. resection will not remove all the cancerous tissue present) means curative procedure unlikely to be successful
    - Primary tumour surrounds the superior mesenteric vein, which is an important blood vessel, and therefore resection ie likely to be impossible without causing damage to this
    - High surgical risk due to deranged LFTs
    - Unclear margins

08. **Delay in diagnosis:** delayed presentation: patient waited 8 weeks to consult (and pancreatic cancer often only causes symptoms at later stage)

Chapter

RENAL AND GENITOURINARY

CASE 1

SCENARIO

A 67-year-old man presents complaining of haematuria, right flank pain, weight loss and pyrexia over the past 3 days. On examination, a palpable mass is found in the right loin, raising suspicion of renal cell carcinoma.

01. Describe the possible mechanisms that could lead to these symptoms.

COMPLETE CDM KEY

02. What 2 diagnostic investigations would you do and why?

03. On the ward round the registrar is doing some teaching and he asks you to name the unique route of direct spread in renal cell carcinoma.

04. The patient goes on to have investigations for staging. Define staging and state its importance.

COMPLETE CDM KEY

RENAL AND GENITOURINARY

CASE 2

SCENARIO

A 66-year-old diabetic patient comes to see you as he has been feeling lethargic, breathless and generally unwell recently. He feels like he is constantly itching and he makes several trips to the toilet each night to urinate. His BP is 151/92mmHg. You think he may have chronic renal failure.

01. Excluding diabetes name 3 other causes of chronic renal failure.

02. Give 2 routine clinical investigations you would do and explain why each would be useful.

COMPLETE CDM KEY

03. What further investigation would you request to assess the severity of chronic renal failure?

04. Give 2 therapeutic measures for managing the patient's symptoms.

A few months later the patient returns to the renal clinic and there has been a marked deterioration. You think that he may need renal replacement therapy.

05. Name 2 examples of temporary renal replacement therapy and list one advantage and on disadvantage for each.

COMPLETE CDM KEY

RENAL AND GENITOURINARY

CASE 3

SCENARIO

A 45-year-old woman with known systemic lupus erythematosus (SLE) presents with pedal oedema. Urinalysis reveals proteinuria. You consider nephrotic syndrome.

01. What 2 laboratory results would confirm the clinical diagnosis of nephrotic syndrome? Provide values.

02. The renal consultant wants to do a renal biopsy and he asks you to check 3 investigations before performing the biopsy-what are they?

03. Give 2 complications of renal biopsy.

04. What is the most likely histological diagnosis in this case?

05. Give 2 autoantibodies that are most commonly detected in SLE.

RENAL AND GENITOURINARY

CASE 4

SCENARIO

You examine a 54-year-old man who has a family history of renal failure. You note that he has palpably enlarged kidneys.

01. What 2 investigations would you order to confirm the abnormality?

02. The consultant makes a provisional diagnosis of polycystic kidneys and she asks you the mode of inheritance.

Bloods show that your patient is anaemic and has features of hyperparathyroidism secondary to his renal failure.

03. Name 1 drug used for each of these 2 complications of renal failure.

COMPLETE CDM KEY

04. Name 2 non-renal complications that are more common in patients with adult polycystic kidneys than the general population.

The patient has been doing some research on the internet and asks you about renal replacement therapy.

05. Give 3 forms of renal replacement therapy that could be discussed with the patient.

COMPLETE CDM KEY

This patient is concerned about his family's risk of developing the disease. He has 2 grandsons (aged 14 and 11) and he asks you whether they should be screened for the condition.

06. What advice would you give?
_____

_____

COMPLETE CDM KEY

RENAL AND GENITOURINARY

CASE 5

SCENARIO

A 79-year-old woman is admitted with acute confusion. She is unable to give any coherent history.

01. Name 3 vitamin deficiencies that can cause acute confusion.

Her daughter is called and when she arrives she tells you that the patient has complained of increased urinary frequency, suprapubic discomfort and new urinary incontinence. You suspect she has a UTI.

02. Give 4 findings that would suggest this from the urine dipstick.

COMPLETE CDM KEY

03. What is the most common organism to cause UTIs in the community?

04. You decide to start an antibiotic; she has normal renal function and a normal urinary tract. What do you prescribe?

When the patient improves, you discuss ways to reduce the recurrence of UTI.

05. What 2 pieces of advice would you give?

COMPLETE CDM KEY

RENAL AND GENITOURINARY

ANSWERS:

Case 1: Renal Cell carcinoma

01. **Mechanism of symptoms:**

    - Haematuria: direct bleeding of the cancer; cancer in the collecting system
    - Right flank pain: stretching of renal capsule caused by cancer; invasion of surrounding structures
    - Weight loss: increased energy demands from rapidly growing cancer; paraneoplastic syndrome
    - Pyrexia: cytokine release from tumour

02. **Investigations:**

    - Urinalysis: microscopy (with cytology for malignant cells)
    - Ultrasound: demonstrate the solid lesion and examine the patency of the renal vein and inferior vena cava
    - CT (guided biopsy)

03. **Direct spread of renal cell carcinoma:** invasion of renal vein to inferior vena cava

04. **Staging:**

    - Staging is the assessment of the extent of disease and is therefore of prognostic significance
    - Uses the TNM classification to consider the tumour (T) size, whether lymph nodes (N) are involved, and whether there are any metastases (M)

Case 2: Chronic renal failure

01. **Causes of chronic renal failure:**

    - Renovascular disease, e.g. renal artery stenosis, hypertension
    - Glomerulonephritis, e.g. idiopathic IgA, lupus nephritis
    - Autosomal dominant polycystic kidney disease (ADPKD)
    - Chronic pyelonephritis
    - Drugs causing renal papillary necrosis, e.g. NSAIDs causing analgesic nehphropathy
    - Chronic obstruction (e.g. pelvic tumour, prostatic hypertrophy / cancer)

02. **Investigations:**

    - U&Es: assess kidney function (elevated urea and creatinine and reduced eGFR with chronic renal failure), possible hyperkalaemia (may require treatment)
    - FBC: the patient displays symptoms of anaemia which is associated with chronic renal failure (anaemia of chronic disease) and may require treatment (erythropoietin (EPO))
    - Urine dipstick: proteinuria (degree of glomerular disease / damage and renal failure), glycosuria (may indicate hyperglycaemia), haematuria / red cell casts (may suggest glomerulonephritis)

03. **Further investigations:**

    - Renal tract ultrasound
    - Albumin: creatinine ratio

04. **Symptomatic management:**

    - Treat anaemia (lethargic, breathless) – exclude iron deficiency anaemia and if it's anaemia of chronic disease consider EPO
    - Treat itch (uraemic pruritus) – emollients and antihistamines

05. **Renal replacement therapy:**
    - **Haemodialysis:**
        - Advantages: faster than peritoneal dialysis (fewer days / weeks) and more effective
        - Disadvantages: disequilibrium syndrome (neurological deterioration); hypotension; increased cardiovascular risk; time-consuming (multiple visits to dialysis centre per week); access is via fistula – risk of thrombosis, stenosis and aneurysm
    - **Peritoneal dialysis:**
        - Advantages: simple to perform; less complex equipment; more freedom (at home so don't need to go to dialysis centre)
        - Disadvantages: peritonitis; exit-site infection; catheter malfunction loss of membrane function; hernias; back pain
    - **Haemofiltration:** blood filtered continuously across a highly permeable synthetic membrane, waste products removed by convection (not diffusion)
        - Advantage: less haemodynamic instability (used for critically ill patients)
        - Disadvantages: expensive; takes longer than haemodialysis.

COMPLETE CDM KEY

Case 3: Nephrotic syndrome

01. **Nephrotic syndrome – triad of oedema:**

    - Serum albumin <30g/L
    - Proteinuria >3g/24h (remember to dip the urine in oedematous patients!)

02. **Pre-biopsy investigations:**

    - **Coagulation screen** (rules out coagulopathy), also U&Es and group and save
    - **Blood pressure** (renal biopsy contraindicated if> 160/90)
    - Renal **ultrasound** (biopsy contraindicated when kidneys <60% predicted size or <9cm due to chronic renal failure; single functioning kidney)

03. **Complications of biopsy:**

    - Haemorrhage: blood loss requiring transfusion in 1-2%
    - Macroscopic haematuria in 10%

04. **Histology in this case:** membranous nephropathy – associated with nephrotic syndrome in SLE

05. **Autoantibodies:**

    - Antinuclear antibodies (ANAs) (not specific to SLE, but present in >95% of patients)
    - ds-DNA antibody (specific to SLE, present in 60% of patients)

COMPLETE CDM KEY

Case 4: Polycystic kidneys

01. **Investigations:**
    - Abdominal ultrasound
    - CT abdomen / pelvis

02. **Mode of inheritance in polycystic kidney disease:** autosomal dominant

    - **Coagulation screen** (rules out coagulopathy), also U&Es and group and save
    - **Blood pressure** (renal biopsy contraindicated if > 160/90)
    - Renal **ultrasound** (biopsy contraindicated when kidneys <60% predicted size or <9cm due to chronic renal failure; single functioning kidney)

03. **Complications of biopsy:**
    - Haemorrhage: blood loss requiring transfusion in 1-2%
    - Macroscopic haematuria in 10%

04. **Histology in this case:** membranous nephropathy – associated with nephrotic syndrome in SLE

05. **Autoantibodies:**
    - Antinuclear antibodies (ANAs) (not specific to SLE, but present in >95% of patients)
    - ds-DNA antibody (specific to SLE, present in 60% of patients)

COMPLETE CDM KEY

Case 5: Urinary tract infection

01. **Vitamin deficiencies causing confusion:**
    - Thiamine (vitamin B1)- Beriberl; Wernicke- Korsakoff's syndrome
    - Niacin (vitamin B3) – pellagra – 3Ds-dermatitis, diarrhoea, dementia
    - Vitamin B12 (hydroxycobalamin)

02. **UTI:** positive dipstick for:
    - Leucocytes
    - Nitrates
    - Protein
    - Red blood cells

03. **Most common community bacteria in UTI =** Escherichia coli

04. **First –choice oral antibiotic in UTI:** trimethoprim

05. **General advice in UTI:**
    - Drink plenty of fluids (2L/day)
    - Practise good hygiene –'wipe front to back'
    - Empty the bladder regularly

CHAPTER

ENDOCRINOLOGY

CASE 1

SCENARIO

A 30-year-old woman presents after finding a swelling in the right side of her neck. A 2cm nodule in the left upper lobe of her thyroid gland is palpable during examination. She mentions that she has lost over a stone in weight over the last 2 months. You think she has thyrotoxicosis.

01. Give 6 other signs would you look for on examination.

COMPLETE CDM KEY

02. What blood tests would you do to confirm the diagnosis?

03. Before starting treatment, what investigations would you do?

04. If she does have thyrotoxicosis, suggest 2 treatments.

COMPLETE CDM KEY

ENDOCRINOLOGY

CASE 2

SCENARIO

You are an FY2 doing a rotation in general practice. You see an 18-year-old man who complains of fatigue. Further questioning reveals that he has increased urinary frequency and has lost 5kg in the last 8 weeks. You think he may have diabetes mellitus.

01. List 3 other questions you would ask him in order to support your provisional diagnosis.

After discussion with the diabetes consultant, the patient is commenced on insulin. As part of your plan, you counsel him on factors that precipitate hypoglycaemia.

02. List 3 factors of which he should be aware.

COMPLETE CDM KEY

03. Give 2 symptoms of hypoglycaemia of which he should be aware.

04. Give 2 therapeutic methods of reducing the chance of this patient developing diabetic nephropathy.

COMPLETE CDM KEY

ENDOCRINOLOGY

CASE 3

SCENARIO

A 42-year-old woman visits you in clinic complaining of weight loss, sweating and palpitations. On examination, you think there is a small smooth goitre. Bloods show a T4 of 68μmol/L (reference range 5-15 μmol/L) and TSH <0.01 μmol/L (reference range 0.2-5 μmol/L).

01. What is the most likely cause for her symptoms and blood results?

02. Name 5 other sings you would look for on clinical examination.

COMPLETE CDM KEY

03. The patient has a visible tremor and you prescribe propranolol. What else would you offer for medical management and what treatment duration would recommend?

04. What options are available for definitive management?

ENDOCRINOLOGY

CASE 4

SCENARIO

You see a 60-year-old man at the diabetic clinic. He was diagnosed with type 2 diabetes 10 years ago. His only complaint is a burning sensation in his feet.

01. How would you assess his long-term glucose control?

In addition to burning in his feet, he also complains of a tingling sensation.

02. What has caused this?

03. He asks you how much more likely it is that he will have a heart attack compared to a non-diabetic man of the same age – what do you say?

COMPLETE CDM KEY

18 months later the patient presents to A&E with double vision. Examination reveals a dilated right pupil. He has diplopia on looking up and to the right.

04. What has happened?

05. Give 4 causes of hypoglycaemia.

COMPLETE CDM KEY

ENDOCRINOLOGY

CASE 5

SCENARIO

A 56-year-old woman who has type 1 diabetes presents to the A&E department with a 2-day history of pain and swelling in her left leg. The patient is confused, with a red, swollen and tender leg, and her breath smells ketotic.

01. Give 3 investigations you would arrange as part of your immediate management plan.

02. Why are diabetic patients prone to complications in their feet?

COMPLETE CDM KEY

03. Name 3 specific sites/ sources you would check for infection.

04. You start the patient on antibiotics, but what two other aspects of the immediate management of this women's diabetes are important?

At the end of your shift, you re-examine the patient. She is complaining of increased pain on the sole of her foot, with marked tenderness and erythema spreading up her calf. You call a senior for advice.

COMPLETE CDM KEY

05. Give 2 possible treatment options.

ENDOCRINOLOGY

CASE 6

SCENARIO

A normally fit 15-year-old boy presents to A&E generally unwell and drowsy. His parents tell you he had a chest infection recently. On examination, he looks unwell dehydrated and he is difficult to rouse. His heart rate is 120bpm and his BP is 95/40mmHg. His abdomen is generally tender. You do an ABG:

- PO_2 12.0kPa
- PCO_2 2.3kPa
- H^+ 101nmol/L
- HCO_3^- 5mmol/L
- Glucose   >50mmol/L

01. What is the most likely diagnosis?

02. What is your immediate management plan?

ENDOCRINOLOGY

ANSWERS

Case 1: Thyrotoxicosis
01. **Clinical features in hyperthyroidism:**

- Warm, sweaty palms
- Thyroid eye disease: exophthalmos, lid retraction, lid lag
- Pretibial myxoedema
- Thyroid bruit
- Palmar erythema
- Fine tremor
- Hair thnning / loss
- Cardiovascular: tachycardia, irregularly irregular pulse (secondary to atrial fibrillation)

- Neurological : decreased power in proximal muscle groups, hyper-reflexia
- Anxiety / restlessness / irritability

Other features which may be in the history include diarrhoea, increased appetite, menorrhagia, infertility, reduced libido, heat intolerance.

02. **Blood tests:**

- TFTs: free T3, T4 increased; serum TSH decreased
- Anti-thyroid antibodies: Anti-thyroid peroxidase (anti-TPO) antibodies, anti-thyroglobulin antibodies, TSH receptor antibodies

03. **Investigations:**

- Thyroid ultrasound and fine needle aspiration
- Radio-iodine uptake scan (to identify 'hot' regions of over activity)
- ECG (may show atrial fibrillation)

04. **Treatment:**

- Radioactive iodine therapy (in non-pregnant, non-lactating patients)
- Nodular goiters are not associated with remission of symptoms after carbimazole therapy (unlike graves' disease)
- Patients may prefer to avoid surgery as far as possible due to its implications (e.g. general anaesthetic) and risk of complications

Case 2: Diabetes mellitus

01. **History in diabetes mellitus:**

- Has he been drinking more than usual? (polydipsia)
- Has he been walking up at night to pass urine? (nocturia)
- Does he have a family history of diabetes or personal history of other autoimmune disease? (e.g. pernicious anaemia, Addison's disease)
- Associated symptoms of hyperglycaemia: has he had any blurred vision, thrush, lethargy?

02. **Factors that precipitate hypoglycaemia:**

- Increased / unexpected exercise
- Skipping meals / dieting
- Alcohol

Intercurrent illness causes hyperglycaemia – type 1 diabetics should still take their insulin to prevent diabetic ketoacidosis (DKA).

03. **Symptoms of hypoglycaemia:**

- **Autonomic:** sweating, anxiety, hunger, tremor, palpitations
- **Neuroglycopenic:** confusion, drowsiness, inability to concentrate, speech difficulty, incoordination, seizures, coma
- Other: nausea, headache, tiredness

04. **Reducing long-term complications:**

- **Maintain good glycaemic control (aim for HbA1c<48mmol/mol):** patient education lifestyle, diet and need for medication compliance; regular home monitoring of blood glucose and adjustment of insulin as necessary
- Regular checks at **diabetic clinic** (BP, cholesterol, urinalysis HbA1c, U&E, retinal screening and neurology checks): treat **hypertension** early (aim for <130/80mmHg) with ACE inhibitors, screen for microscopic albuminuria and start on ACE inhibitor if detected regardless of BP

Case 3: Primary hyperthyroidism

01. **Diagnosis:** primary hyperthyroidism

02. **Clinical features:**
    - Warm, sweaty palms
    - Thyroid eye disease: exophthalmos, lid retraction, lid lag
    - Pretibial myxedema
    - Thyroid bruit
    - Palmar erythema
    - Fine tremor
    - Hair thinning / loss
    - Cardiovascular: tachycardia, irregularly irregular pulse (secondary to atrial fibrillation)
    - Neurological: decreased power in proximal muscle groups, hyper-reflexia

03. **Medical treatment of thyrotoxicosis:**
    - Titration to TFTs: carbimazole / propylthiouracil (PTU)
    - Block and replace: carbimazole and thyroxine
    - Duration: 12-18 months

04. **Other treatment:**
    - Radio-iodine therapy
    - Subtotal or total thyroidectomy

COMPLETE CDM KEY

Case 4: Type 2 diabetes

01. **Assessing glucose control:**

    - Diary of finger stick glucose records
    - Glycated haemoglobin (HbA1c)

02. **Burning and tingling in a diabetic:**

    - **Peripheral neuropathy**
    - Hyperglycaemia produces end-glycation products which cause dysfunction of nerves leading to paraesthesia (i.e. neuropathy)
    - This effects the most distal nerves first in a 'glove and stocking' pattern, therefore his feet are the most symptomatic

03. **Cardiovascular risk:** 3-5 more likely to encounter cardiovascular complications than a non-diabetic

04. **Dilated pupil and diplopia looking up and to the right in diabetes:** mononeuropathy of the oculomotor nerve (CNIII) as a result of chronic hyperglycaemia

05. **Causes of hypoglycaemia:**

    - Exogenous drugs: insulin, sulphonylureas, alcohol
    - In a diabetic: skipped meals / strict dieting, unexpected exercise
    - In a non-diabetic: pituitary insufficiency, liver failure, adrenal insufficiency (e.g. addison's disease), insulinoma, non-pancreatic neoplasms (e.g. retroperitoneal fibrosarcoma)

COMPLETE CDM KEY

Case 5: Type 2 diabetes

01. **Assessing glucose control:**

    - Diary of finger stick glucose records
    - Glycated haemoglobin (HbA1c)

02. **Burning and tingling in a diabetic:**

    - **Peripheral neuropathy**
    - Hyperglycaemia produces end-glycation products which cause dysfunction of nerves leading to paraesthesia (i.e. neuropathy)
    - This effects the most distal nerves first in a 'glove and stocking' pattern, therefore his feet are the most symptomatic

03. **Cardiovascular risk:** 3-5 more likely to encounter cardiovascular complications than a non-diabetic

04. **Dilated pupil and diplopia looking up and to the right in diabetes:** mononeuropathy of the oculomotor nerve (CNIII) as a result of chronic hyperglycaemia

05. **Causes of hypoglycaemia:**

    - Exogenous drugs: insulin, sulphonylureas, alcohol
    - In a diabetic: skipped meals / strict dieting, unexpected exercise
    - In a non-diabetic: pituitary insufficiency, liver failure, adrenal insufficiency (e.g. addison's disease), insulinoma, non-pancreatic neoplasms (e.g. retroperitoneal fibrosarcoma)

COMPLETE CDM KEY

Case 6: Type 1 diabetes

01. **Investigations:**

    - Bloods – FBC; U&Es; LFTs; CRP; serum glucose
    - ABG – look for sings of DKA
    - Urine dipstick

02. **Pathophysiology of diabetic foot:**

    - Hyperglycaemia leads to macro-and microvascular disease which can lead to peripheral vascular disease, therefore decreasing tissue perfusion of the feet; this leads to trophic and ischaemeic changes, poor healing, and ulceration especially over pressure areas.
    - Hyperglycaemia causes peripheral neuropathy which leads to decreased sensation in the feet ('glove and stocking' pattern) and this makes incidental injury more likely due to loss of tactile sensation and proprioception which may lead to open sores that can become infected

03. **Portals of infection:**

    - **Skin:** look for cuts / fissures / ulcers on feet (including between the toes) and legs, subcutaneous injection sites
    - **IV cannulation sites:** swab / blood culture
    - **Urinary tract:** check with urine dipstick, analysis and culture

04. **Further management of unwell type 1 diabetic:**

    - **Monitoring:** ABCDE approach; GCS; blood glucose; U&Es (especially K^+), HCO_3^-; urine output; ketones; vital signs
    - **Insulin administration and fluid / potassium replacement:** for insulin aim for a fall in glucose of 5mmol/h with sliding scale; should initially give 0.9% saline, then 5% dextrose once glucose is <15mmol/L; if in DKA – use local DKA protocol

05. **If deteriorating / not improving:**

    - Surgery: exploration, debridement and washout
    - Check antibiotic sensitivity and change antibiotic (use stronger broad-spectrum antibiotic given as a high dose intravenously)

COMPLETE CDM KEY

Case 7: Diabetic ketoacidosis

01. **Drowsy + unwell + hyperglycaemia + metabolic acidosis =** diabetic ketoacidosis (DKA)

02. **Immediate management:**

- ABCDE approach and call senior for help
- Secure airway and start high flow oxygen via trauma mask
- Gain IV access with 2 wide-bore cannula and take bloods: glucose, FBC, U&Es, bicarb, culture, toxicology screen, ABG
- Start IV fluids immediately; 0.9% saline with replacement of K+ later guided by U&Es; 5% dextrose once glucose <15mmol/L 1 Lover next hour, 1L over the next 2h, 1L over the next 4h
- Give 4-8 units insulin stat if plasma glucose >20mmol/L. 1L stat, 1L on sliding scale (aim to reduce by 5mmol/h)-DKA protocol
- Monitor vital signs, consciousness level, urine output and ketones; insert catheter if no urine passed for >4h
- Give heparin SC until mobile (VTE risk)
- Find and treat infection

CHAPTER

NEUROLOGY

CASE 1

SCENARIO

A 69-year old man comes to see you with a new tremor. He finds it difficult to start walking and he has been falling recently. His wife says he is generally slower in his daily activities. You suspect idiopathic Parkinson's disease.

COMPLETE CDM KEY

01. Which clinical features of Parkinson's disease comprise a classical triad? Suggest a feature of each that you would expect to see on examination.

02. What sensory signs would you expect to see in Parkinson's disease?

03. Explain how the pathological process in the brain results in the clinical features.

COMPLETE CDM KEY

You discuss the patient with your supervisor and they advise that Parkinson's disease can be classified as an akinetic-rigid syndrome.

04. They ask you to name 3 other example of akinetic-rigid syndrome.

05. What is the difference between parkinsonism and idiopathic Parkinson's disease?

06. Your consultant wants to start treatment. Give 2 classes of drugs used in the treatment of Parkinson's disease and describe their mechanism of action.

COMPLETE CDM KEY

07. Draw a synapse and mark on the figure where the 2 drugs act.

08. What issues should be considered when using drug therapies for the treatment of Parkinson's disease?

08. What psychiatric illness is common following diagnosis in patients suffering from Parkinson's disease and what drug may be used to treat this?

NEUROLOGY

CASE 2

SCENARIO

An 85-year-old man is found collapsed on the living room floor by his carer. He is noted to have a significant weakness on the left side of his body. He is confused and disorientated.

01. You suspect he has had a stroke. How would you define stroke?

02. Give 4 risk factors for a stroke.

COMPLETE CDM KEY

You organize a CT head which reveals an area of ischaemia.

03. Explain the pathogenesis of this type of stroke.

04. In terms of this patient's symptoms, which blood vessel in the brain has likely been affected?.

COMPLETE CDM KEY

05. Name 6 significant complications of stroke.

NEUROLOGY

CASE 3

SCENARIO

You are called to A&E to see a 32-year-old man who has been brought in by ambulance with a short history of severe, sudden onset, occipital headache. He is normally fit and well. He is now unconscious and his breathing is laboured.

01. What scoring system would you use to quantify the level of consciousness?

02. What conditions would you suspect to be the cause of his problem?

03. What investigation would you request to confirm the diagnosis?

COMPLETE CDM KEY

04. The consultant asks you to perform a lumbar puncture. What may be precipitated by this procedure?

The patient is admitted ITU but unfortunately, he makes no signs of recovery and brainstem death is confirmed. He has an organ donor card in his wallet.

05. Give 2 medical conditions that would preclude organ donation.

06. What 2 key points should be covered when you speak with the patient's family about brainstem death?

NEUROLOGY

CASE 4

SCENARIO

A 70-year-old man brought to A&E by ambulance having been discovered on his kitchen floor by his daughter. On examination he is obese, mumbling, pale and drowsy. He is hypothermic with a rectal temperature of 31°C. Heart rate is 51bpm and BP is 100/50mmHg. His daughter has brought his medication including levothyroxine, gliclazide, paracetamol and prednisolone (5mg/day).

01. What are your top 4 differential diagnoses?

02. What is your immediate management?

COMPLETE CDM KEY

03. What important observations would you ask the nurse to monitor?

He is found to be anaemic with a haemoglobin of 7.1g/dl and MCV of 112fl.

04. Give the 3 most likely causes to account for this.

COMPLETE CDM KEY

NEUROLOGY

CASE 5

SCENARIO

You are an FY2 in paediatric emergency medicine. The standby phone goes of: the paramedics are bringing in a 15-year-old boy with known epilepsy. He has been seizing for more than 35 minutes.

01. What is your provisional diagnosis?

When the ambulance arrives, the patient's father states that his son is poorly compliant with medication.

02. Give 3 other possible causes for his presentation.

COMPLETE CDM KEY

03. The registrar asks you to again IV access immediately and send off urgent bloods. Suggest 3 important tests in this patient.

04. What 2 immediate treatments will you institute?

Despite your best efforts, the patient continues to fit. The registrar asks the nurse to start an IV infusion.

05. What does the infusion contain?

COMPLETE CDM KEY

COMPLETE CDM KEY

NEUROLOGY

ANSWERS

Case 1: **Parkinson's disease**

01. **Parkinson's triad:**

- Tremor
  - Most marked at rest; typically 'pill rolling'; 4-6Hz
- Rigidity
  - Lead pipe – increased resistance to passive stretch of muscles throughout range of movement
  - Cog-wheel – tone may be broken up by tremor
- Bradykinesia
  - Slowed initiation of movements

Other features of note include postural instability, monotonous speech, loss of facial expression, reduced blink reflex, micrographia and shuffling gait.

02. **Sensory disturbance in Parkinson's:** anosmia

03. **Pathophysiology of Parkinson's:**

Degeneration and loss of dopaminergic neurons in the substantia nigra of the basal ganglia leads to decreased dopamine transmission in the nigrostriatal pathway. This means there is an imbalance between the amount of acetylcholine and dopamine. The direct pathway responsible for initiating movement is inhibited and the indirect pathway which inhibits movements is excited. When

60-80% of dopaminergic neurons are lost, extrapyramidal signs and symptoms appear such as tremor, rigidity and bradykinesia.

04. **Akinetic-rigid syndromes:**

- Drug-induced parkinsonism (e.g. sodium valproate, metoclopramide, prochlorperazine)
- Post- encephalitic Parkinsonism
- Progressive supranuclear palsy
- Multiple system atrophy

05. **Parkinsonism vs. Parkinson's disease:**

- Parkinsonism – term used to describe the clinical features of tremor, rigidity and bradykinesia regardless of aetiology; it is seen in Parkinson's disease but is not exclusive to it.
- Idiopathic Parkinson's disease – a condition that present with the features of parkinsonism but specifically with idiopathic loss of dopaminergic neurons in the substantia nigra

06. **Centrally acting treatment:**

- **Levodopa** (often given alongside decarboxylase inhibitors such as carbidopa to reduce peripheral side effects of systemic dopamine such as nausea) this is a dopamine precursor which is able to cross the blood – brain barrier and be converted to dopamine where it can agonise dopamine receptors
- **Dopamine receptor agonists** (such as bromocriptine, cabergoline and ropinirole) act directly on dopamine receptors principally D1 and D2 receptors; this enhances dopaminergic action at receptors
- **Catechol-o-methyltransferase (COMT) inhibitors** (such as entacapone) block the action of COMT-the enzyme responsible for the brackdown of dopamine once in the synapse
- **Monoamine oxidase B (MAO-B) inhibitors** (such as selegiline) block the action of MAO-B-the enzyme responsible for the

breakdown of dopamine before it reaches the synapse; as with COMT inhibitors, these drugs also prolong the dopaminergic effect.

07.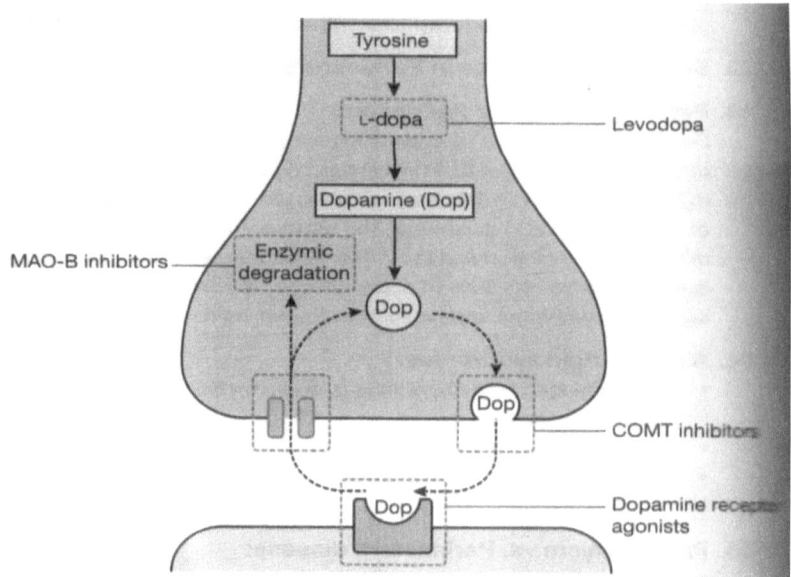

08. **Medication considerations**

    - Side-effects, e.g. hallucination, dizziness, nausea, addiction, gambling
    - Problems associated with prolonged or high dose L-dopa include motor fluctuations (end of dose effect, on/off effect) and dyskinesia (peak dose, diphasic, dystonia)
    - Patient age and severity of their symptoms is important because with longer life expectancy it is advised to delay L-dopa; this is due to drug side-effects becoming more pronounced after 10 years of use

COMPLETE CDM KEY

09. **Psychiatric:** depression occurs in approximately 50% of cases and is most effectively treated using selective serotonin reuptake inhibitors (SSRIs)

Case 2: Stroke

01. **Stroke definition:** a stroke is a rapidly developing focal neurological deficit of presumed vascular origin lasting more than 24 hours or causing death.

02. **Stroke risks:** hypertension, diabetes mellitus, atrial fibrillation, smoking, previous TIA or stroke, hypercholesterolaemia

03. **Pathophysiology of ischaemic stroke:**

    Decreased blood flow in one of the cerebral arteries (usually due to thrombus formation on an unstable atherosclerotic plaque in carotid or vertebral artery, or an embolus from a downstream thrombus) causes decreased perfusion of the area of brain tissue which it supplies. As the brain has a high demand for oxygen and glucose this area ceases to function rapidly and there is cellular injury. This leads to glutamate excitotoxicity, causing nearby cells to undergo similar changes due to glutamine and calcium efflux. Grossly there is an area of tissue necrosis, often with an ischaemic penumbra and surrounding oedema. There may be cerebral effacement and midline shift in large ischaemic strokes.

04. **Left-sided weakness:** right middle cerebral artery

05. **Complications of stroke:**

    - Depression
    - Aspiration which may lead to pneumonia
    - Immobility which can lead to pressure sores
    - Urinary incontinence
    - Communication difficulty from dysphasia
    - Venous thromboembolism

Case 3: Brainstem death

01. **assessing neurological insult:** Glasgow coma Scale (GCS)

02. **Differential diagnosis:**
    - Subarachnoid haemorrhage
    - Meningitis
    - Space-occupying lesion, such as tumour or abscess
    - Cerebral trauma

03. **Investigation:** CT head

04. **Lumber puncture + raised intracranial pressure** = coning = herniation of the cerebellar tonsils through the foramen magnum due to increased intracranial pressure

05. **Contraindications to organ donation:**
    - Infections such as HIV and CJD
    - Malignancy

06. **Talking to relative about brainstem death:**
    - The patient is deeply unconscious and there is cessation of the most basic functions of the brain (brainstem functions)
    - This is due to irreversible brain damage and there is no evidence that this state may have been caused by a correctable abnormality
    - The person is unable to breath spontaneously and therefore their life is being maintained solely by the ventilator and other supportive treatment
    - In this state their heart will stop beating in a few days despite ventilation and so it is humane to withdraw 'life support'
    - Brainstem death is confirmed by two different medical practitioners on separate occasions

COMPLETE CDM KEY

Case 4: Unconscious patient

01. **Differential diagnosis:**
    - Myxedema crisis (on thyroxine – severe hypothyroidism)
    - Addisonian crisis (on long-term prednisolone – think acute adrenal insufficiency)
    - Hypoglycaemia or hyperosmolar hyperglycaemic state (HHS) (on gliclazide)
    - Stroke

02. **Immediate management:**
    - Gain IV access for taking bloods (FBC, U&Es, LFTs, CRP, TFTs, glucose) and give IV fluids
    - IV hydrocortisone and IV thyroid replacement
    - Rewarming using bear hugger / blankets / warm fluids

03. **Observations:**
    - Level of consciousness (GCS)
    - Oxygen saturations
    - Temperature
    - HR and blood pressure

04. **Macrocytic anaemia:**
    - Severe hypothyroidism
    - Alcohol abuse
    - Vitamin B12 and folate deficiency

COMPLETE CDM KEY

Case 5: Epilepsy

01. **Diagnosis:** status epilepticus

02. **Precipitating factors:**
    - Alcohol
    - Illicit drugs
    - Infection inadequate anti-epileptic drug dose

03. **Investigations:**
    - Urea and electrolytes
    - Full blood count
    - Glucose
    - Liver function tests
    - Toxicology
    - Anticonvulsant levels (if appropriate)

04. **Management:**
    - 100% oxygen via a trauma mask
    - IV benzodiazepine, e.g. lorazepam

05. **if seizure continues despite benzodiazepine, consider:** IV phenytoin infusion (18mg/Kg)

CHAPTER

RHEUMATOLOGY

CASE 1

SCENARIO

A 45-year-old woman complains of pain in her hands and wrists for the past 8 months. In addition, she reports that her eyes have been painful, red and watery for 8 days now and they are sore to touch. You suspect that she has rehmatoid arthritis. You request an X-ray of her hand sendoff bloods.

01. What X-ray features would support your clinical suspicion of rheumatoid arthritis?

_____

_____

_____

The patient's routine blood results reveal raised CRP and reduced haemogobin.

02. Provide an explanation for each of these results.

You think that rheumatoid disease is the most likely cause for her eye problems.

03. Give 2 ophthalmic complications that are linked to rheumatoid arthritis.

COMPLETE CDM KEY

The care of patients with rheumatoid arthritis relies on a multi-disciplinary approach.

04. Other than the GP and rheumatologist, name 3 other health professionals that may assist in the management of this patient's chronic illness and describe what they would each contribute.

RHEUMATOLOGY

CASE 2

SCENARIO

A 66-year-old woman complains of progressively worsening pain in the left groin and left knee. The pain peaks in intensity when she walks, and in the evening. The patient has a BMI of 4.

01. Name the joint involved and indicate the most likely diagnosis.

02. You send the patient for an X-ray list 4 features that you would expect to see to support your diagnosis.

03. How would you manage this patient? Outline 2 aspects of management and indicate which one you think is most important.

COMPLETE CDM KEY

04. Eight months later, the patient presents with pain that is now walking her up at night. What procedure might be indicated now?

05. The patient asks about the long-term complications of this procedure – describe 2 long –term complications that are important to discuss.

COMPLETE CDM KEY

COMPLETE CDM KEY

RHEUMATOLOGY

CASE 3

SCENARIO

A 47-year-old woman presents with a burning pain in her left hand that shoots up her arm. It is worse at night. You think that she may have carpal tunnel syndrome.

01. What other symptoms would you enquire about to support your provisional diagnosis?

02. Give 4 clinical features that would support a diagnosis of carpal tunnel syndrome.

COMPLETE CDM KEY

03. List 6 conditions that are associated with carpal tunnel syndrome.

___

___

___

___

___

___

04. How would you manage carpal tunnel syndrome?

___

___

___

05. You are the FY2 in an orthopedic outpatient clinic and the consultant is giving some informal teaching. He asks you to give 2 symptoms and signs of ulnar never entrapment that differentials it from carpal tunnel syndrome.

___

___

___

___

RHEUMATOLOGY

CASE 4

SCENARIO

A 36-year-old man presents to his GP with a history of gradual onset of pain, stiffness and swelling in both of his hands. The symptoms are worse in the morning. He has a strong family history of rheumatoid arthritis. The GP sends a request for bloods, including rheumatoid factor, which has come back elevated.

01. What 2 questions would you like to ask in the history to support a diagnosis of rheumatoid arthritis?

02. Rheumatoid arthritis (RA) has a genetic component. What is the HLA type associated with RA?

03. When you examine his hands you think there are boutonnlere and swan-neck deformities. What leads to these signs?

COMPLETE CDM KEY

As Part of the investigations, the patient has an X-ray.

04. What X-ray features would you expect to see?

The patient is started on a non-steridal anti-inflammatory drug (NSAID)

05. What is the mechanism of action of NSAIDs and give 2 common side-effects?

COMPLETE CDM KEY

Two years later, the patient is seen at rheumatology clinic where he now complains of dry eyes and a dry mouth.

06. What is the likely cause?

   _____

   _____

07. Name 2 other extra-articular manifestations (give 1 haematological and 1 cardiovascular.

   _____

   _____

COMPLETE CDM KEY

RHEUMATOLOGY

CASE 5

SCENARIO

A 63-year-old woman presents with a 4-month history of worsening exertional dyspnea. She was diagnosed with rheumatoid arthritis 20 years ago. On examination she has finger clubbing and fine inspiratory crackles on auscultation of the chest.

01. What signs of rheumatoid disease would you look for in her hands?

COMPLETE CDM KEY

02. Why do you think she has finger clubbing? What investigation would you order to support this?

03. Bloods come back showing she has a haemoglobin of 7.9g/dl. What is the most likely reason for this?

COMPLETE CDM KEY

RHEUMATOLOGY

CASE 6

SCENARIO

A 10-year-old boy presents to A&E with a 2-day history of severe pain and swelling in his right forearm. There is no history of trauma. He is pyrexial. His forearm is tender, hot and erythematous. You suspect osteomyelitis.

01. What 2 investigations would you do to support your provisional diagnosis?

02. Give 2 other causes of a swelling in the forearm that you would include in you differential diagnosis.

03. What is your initial management? Explain your rationale.

COMPLETE CDM KEY

04. The patient is started on treatment and admitted on the ward. How would you monitor his condition?

COMPLETE CDM KEY

RHEUMATOLOGY

CASE 7

SCENARIO

A 65-year-old man with a history of chronic renal failure on dialysis presents with a gradual onset pain and tingling in both his hands. The pain is particularly bad at night.

01. What is your provisional diagnosis?

02. If the diagnosis wasn't clear from history and examination, what investigation could confirm the diagnosis?

03. Give 4 other conditions that can cause this condition.

04. What has been the precipitating cause in this patient?

COMPLETE CDM KEY

05. The patient asks you if there are any long-term complications of dialysis – give 3.

COMPLETE CDM KEY

06. You are the discussing the case with the consultant and are talking about renal transplantation. She asks you to give 2 reasons why renal transplantation would be contraindicated.

COMPLETE CDM KEY

RHEUMATOLOGY

CASE 8

SCENARIO

You are the FY2 in A&E. the standby phone goes off and the paramedics report that they are bringing in an 82-year-old patient who fell at the supermarket. They think he has a fracture neck of femur.

01. Whilst waiting for the ambulance, the registrar asks you to give 4 clinic features that would be in keeping with a fractured neck of femur

_____

_____

_____

_____

_____

_____

_____

_____

02. What information would you want to gain from the history?

COMPLETE CDM KEY

03. What will be your immediate management?

04. What clinical areas will be assessed when the patient arrives in hospital?

COMPLETE CDM KEY

05. Give 3 complications of a fractured neck of femur.

RHEUMATOLOGY

ANSWERS

Case 1: Rheumatoid arthritis

01. **X-ray findings:**

    - Loss of joint space
    - Juxta-articular
    - Soft tissue swelling
    - Juxta-articular osteopenia
    - Joint deformity / subluxation

02. **Bloods:**

    - Raised CRP;
        - In RA, immune complexes stimulate cytokines (IL-1 and IL-6) and complement activation which leads to synovitis
        - This causes the liver to produce CRP, an acute phase protein and sign of inflammation
    - Reduced haemoglobin:
        - Chronic inflammation leads to anaemia of chronic disease
        - The release of pro-inflammatory cytokines (especially IL-6) decreases EPO synthesis form the kidney and impairs iron availability for haematopoiesis

03. **Eye complications of RA:**

    - Sclaritis
    - Episcleritis
    - Keratoconjunctivitis sicca

04. **The MDT:**

- Orthopedic surgeon – may provide prophylaxis / correction of joint destruction and deformity such as:
  - Synovectomy (reduces bulk of inflamed tissue)
  - Tendon surgery for deformity
  - Excision arthroplasty (e.g. ulnar styloid to reduce pain, metatarsal heads)
  - Total joint replacement arthroplasty such as his, knees, shoulders, elbows and fingers
- Physiotherapists-give advice on combination of rest (when active arthritis) and exercises to maintain joint range and muscle power:
  - Dynamic exercise therapy
  - Hydrotherapy
  - Some advice for using a TENS machine
- Occupational therapists:
  - Give advice on washing, toileting, dressing, cooking, eating, working,
  - Provide adaptations and aids for the home to reduce limitations in function and improve independence in daily living activities
  - May implement joint protection with splints, methods to reduce strain, and rest regimes

Case 2: Osteoarthritis

01. **Diagnosis:** osteoarthritis – left hip

02. **X-ray features:**

- Loss of joint space
- Peri-articular osteophytes
- Subchondral cysts
- Subchondral sclerosis

03. **Management:**

- Non-pharmacological management: maintain target BMI, moderate exercise, physiotherapy to maximise joint movement and maximise functional ability, occupational assessment for home adaptations / aids for daily living, supportive footwear
- Pharmacological management: simple analgesics such as paracetamol then NSAIDs (e.g. ibuprofen), intra-articular steroid injections

04. **Surgery:** total hip arthroplasty

05. **Complications:**
    - Most commonly, there may be the need for repeated surgery after several years as the joint gradually loosens with activity
    - There may be late infection of the joint, which would present with increasing pain and stiffness and would require antibiotics in addition to two – stage revision surgery

Case 3: Carpal tunnel syndrome

01. **Symptoms:**
    - Paraesthesia (in median nerve territory: thumb, index finger, middle finger and lateral half of ring finger)
    - Decreased sensation and weakness of abductor pollicis brevis

02. **Signs:**
    - Reduced sensation in median nerve territory
    - Wasting of muscles of thenar eminence
    - Weakness of abduction of thumb (abductor pollicis brevis)
    - Positive phalen's test (reproduces symptoms on full flexion of wrists >1min)
    - Positive tinel's test (paraesthesia on tapping over course of median nerve)

03. **Conditions associated with carpal tunnel syndrome:**

    - Acromegaly
    - Rheumatoid arthritis
    - Pregnancy
    - Trauma
    - Renal dialysis (from AV fistula)
    - Hypothyroidism
    - Diabetes

04. **Management:**

    - Conservative – wrist splint, intra-articular joint injection, avoidance of activities which precipitate pain
    - Decompression surgery – division of flexor retinaculum

05. **Ulnar nerve entrapment:**

    - Distribution of numbness and paraesthesia – medial half of ring finger and little finger
    - Wasting of hypothenar eminence and interossei
    - Weakness of abduction of fingers – can't cross fingers due to weakness of interossei
    - Froment's sing: flexion of PIP joint while grasping piece of paper between thumb and index finger due to weakness of adductor pollicis
    - Weakness of wrist flexors (ulnar side)

COMPLETE CDM KEY

Case 4: Rheumatoid arthritis

01. **Clinical questions:**
    - Is there any pain or stiffness in any other joints?
    - How long does the stiffness last in the morning?
    - Have you had any weakness / fatigue / weight loss / fever?
    - Have you noticed any nodules in your arms / sore eyes / trouble breathing?

02. **HLA in RA** = HLA DR4/DR1

03. **Deformities:**
    - Boutonniere deformity:
        - Dorsal synovitis produces DIP hyperextension, PIP flexion and MCP hyperextension
    - Swan – neck deformity:
        - PIP hyperextension with concurrent DIP flexion
        - Due to synovitis of MCP, PIP, or DIP joints which disrupts the balance between flexion and extension forces acting across the joint

04. **X-ray features:**
    - Loss of joint space
    - Bony erosions
    - Soft tissue swelling
    - Juxta-articular osteopenia

05. **NSAID mechanism of action:**
    - NSAIDs are cyclo-oxygenase inhibitors which inhibit the conversion of arachidonic acid acid to prostaglandins and leukotrienes (inflammatory mediators)
    - Side-effect:
        - Gastritis / gastric ulcers
        - Hypersensitivity – bronchoconstriction
        - Nausea and vomiting
        - Diarrhoea

06. **Joint pain + dry eyes + dry mouth** = Sjogren's syndrome

07. **Extra – articular manifestations:**

- Blood-anaemia of chronic disease, thrombocytosis, eosinophilia, neutropenia (in Felty's syndrome)
- Heart – myocardial inflation (secondary to coronary artery disease), pericardial effusion, coronary vasculitis

Case 5: Rheumatoid arthritis

01. **Hand signs in RA:**

- Ulnar deviation of fingers and dorsal wrist subluxation
- Swan – neck deformity of finger
- Boutonniere deformity of finger
- Z-shaped thumb
- Joint swelling, especially of MCP joints, PIP joints and wrist
- Piano key deformity of wrist

02. **Finger clubbing:**

- RA is associated with pulmonary fibrosis / fibrosing alveolitis
- Investigated via high resolution CT scan

03. **Anaemia in RA:**

- Anaemia of chronic disease – chronic inflammation is associated with the release of cytokines which inhibits EPO secretion from the kidney and decreases iron availability for haematopoiesis, causing normochromic, normocytic anaemia
- May also be due to GI blood loss from chronic use of NSAIDs
- DMARDs used for RA may have the side-effect of marrow toxicity leading to pancytopenia (e.g. methotrexate)

Case 6: Osteomyelitis

01. **Investigating osteomyelitis:**
    - Imaging – X-ray; MRI of forearm
    - Blood cultures

02. **Differential diagnosis:**
    - Cellulitis
    - Ewing's sarcoma / osteosarcoma
    - Trauma (fracture with possible compartment syndrome)

03. **Management:**
    - Analgesia (step-wise approach) – to reduce distress and ease pain (as well as bring down temperature); splint and rest arm
    - Empirical antibiotics – use flucloxacillin until organisms and sensitivities known, to treat infection and prevent bone necrosis / chronic infection
    - Admit and refer to orthopaedic surgeon for possible surgical drainage

04. **Monitoring clinical status:**
    - Repeat clinical examination and monitor vital signs: temperature, HR RR, urine output, BP, O_2 sats and check for improvement of symptoms
    - Blood tests – monitor inflammatory markers
    - Imaging – repeat X-rays

COMPLETE CDM KEY

Case 7: Carpal tunnel syndrome

01. **Diagnosis:** carpal tunnel syndrome

02. **Investigation:** electromyography – nerve conduction studies (decreased nerve conduction in median nerve)

03. **Precipitating conditions:**
    - Diabetes mellitus
    - Hypothyroidism
    - Acromegaly
    - Rheumatoid arthritis
    - Pregnancy

04. **Carpal tunnel syndrome in this patient:** AV fistula (used or haemodialysis) – increased venous pressure causes increased pressure in the carpal tunnel and nerve ischaemia

05. **Long-term complications of renal replacement therapy:**
    - Infection (e.g. central line, peritonitis with CAPD)
    - Cardiovascular disease / heart failure
    - Hypertension
    - Amyloidosis (β_2 immunoglobulin is not filtered during dialysis)
    - Hypotension (due to fluid shifts)
    - Metabolic (hypokalaemia, hyper-/hyponatraemia)
    - Anaemia
    - Bleeding tendency
    - Renal bone disease
    - Acquired renal cysts
    - Malignancy

06. **Contraindications to transplant:**
    - Disseminated malignancy
    - Acute infection
    - Persistent substance abuse
    - Severe heart disease or co-morbidity (hepatic failure)
    - Severe psychiatric disease – relative contraindication

Case 8: Fractured neck of femur

COMPLETE CDM KEY

01. **Fractured neck of femur:**
    - Leg adducted and externally rotated
    - Discrepancy in leg length (shorter on fractured side)
    - All movements are extremely painful
    - Inability to walk / weight bear
    - On palpation, tenderness over the anterior and lateral aspects of the hip
    - The greater trochanter is elevated on the injured side

02. **History:**
    - History of injury
    - Past medical history – significant co-morbidities (e.g. osteoporosis, malignancy)
    - Medication
    - Allergies
    - Social history – who is at home / nearby family / social services support, whether he live in house / flat / supported accommodation, smoking and alcohol status

03. **Immediate management**
    - Assess ABCDE
    - Gain IV access and take bloods including group and save
    - Provide analgesia (IV morphine 5-10mg titrated)
    - X-ray pelvis
    - Consider nerve block (senior support)
    - Splint leg to support it and avoid movement
    - Ensure the patient is kept warm
    - Refer to orthopaedics

04. **Assessment:**
    - Airway, breathing and circulation
    - Mental state-GCS
    - Top-to-toe examination for co-existing injury (e.g. head injury) and for co-morbidities (e.g. heart failure /COPD, nutritional status)
    - Orthopaedic assessment – hip movement, neurovascular integrity (with prompt X-ray of pelvis)
    - Assessment of pain – need for femoral nerve block, morphine
    - Anaesthetic assessment – for potential surgery (with ECG, CXR, bloods – FBC/U&Es/ coagulation screen / cross – match)

05. **Complications:**
- Non-union (leading to arthritis and decreased mobility) / mal-union / delayed union
- Avascular necrosis of femoral head (can lead to collapse)
- Thromboembolism – DVT, PE, stroke
- Worsening of co-morbidities (e.g. heart failure and increased susceptibility to infection such as pneumonia)

CHAPTER

DERMATOLOGY

CASE 1

SCENARIO

You see an 18-year-old man at the dermatology clinic. He has a widespread rash affecting his knees and elbows. There are multiple white plaques in keeping with plaque psoriasis.

01. Give 3 other types of psoriasis.

COMPLETE CDM KEY

02. Name 2 classes of drugs that can exacerbate psoriasis.

03. When you examine his nails, you note some abnormalities. Name 4 nail changes that are seen in psoriasis.

COMPLETE CDM KEY

04. Give 4 examples of treatment that you could commence.

You see the patient 6 months later. Unfortunately, his symptoms are worse and he now has severe psoriasis. You discuss his case with the consultant. She recommends acitretin, an oral retinoid.

05. Who should not get this treatment and why?

COMPLETE CDM KEY

DERMATOLOGY

CASE 2

SCENARIO

A 32-year-old lady presents to her GP with a changing, pigmented lesion on her left shoulder. She has a past medical history of inflammatory arthritis and her only medication is adalimumab. The GP suspects malignant melanoma.

01. How would you assess the lesion?

The GP refers to dermatology and biopsy confirms melanoma.

02. What do you think has contributed to the development of melanoma? Name 4 other risk factors.

COMPLETE CDM KEY

03. Name 4 types of melanoma.

04. How would you determine prognosis?

COMPLETE CDM KEY

DERMATOLOGY

CASE 3

SCENARIO

A 6-year-old boy presents with an itchy rash behind his knees. His mum had a similar rash when she was a child. The GP suspects eczema.

01. What is the pathophysiology of eczema?

02. What is the most common type?

COMPLETE CDM KEY

03. Outline the management options.

04. Give 2 potential complications.

DERMATOLOGY

CASE 4

SCENARIO

A 39-year-old intravenous drug user (IVDU) presents with severe pain, spreading erythema and swelling in her left groin. She looks unwell, with fever and tachycardia. On examination, you think you can feel crepitus over her groin.

01. What diagnosis must be considered?

02. What is the most likely causative organism?

03. What is your immediate management plan?

COMPLETE CDM KEY

COMPLETE CDM KEY

DERMATOLOGY

ANSWERS

Case 1: Psoriasis

01. **Psoriasis:**

    - Guttate psoriasis
    - Flexural psoriasis
    - Erythrodemic psoriasis
    - Pustular psoriasis

02. **Exacerbating drugs:**

    - Beta-blockers
    - Lithium
    - NSAIDs
    - ACE inhibitors

03. **Psoriatic nail changes:**

    - Nail pitting
    - Onycholysis
    - Subungual
    - Yellow / brown discolouration

04. **Treatment**

    - Emollients ($\pm$ salicylic acid)
    - Topical vitamin D preparations, such as calcitriol
    - Topical tar preparations
    - Topical steroids
    - Dithranol cream
    - Retinoids such as tazarotene

05. **Retinoids contraindicated in:** women of childbearing age, because acitretin is teratogenic.

COMPLETE CDM KEY

DERMATOLOGY

Case 2: Malignant melanoma

01. **Assessment of pigmented skin lesions**

    The 'ABCDE Symptoms' criteria represent a method used to evaluate pigmented (melanocytic) skin lesions:

    - **A**symmetrical shape
    - **B**order irregularity
    - **C**olour irregularity
    - **D**iameter >7mm
    - **E**volution of lesion (e.g. change in size or shape)
    - **S**ymptoms (e.g. bleeding, itching)

02. **Risk factors:**

    - Adalimumab (TNF inhibitor) may have contributed to the development of malignant melanoma in this case. Adalimumab is associated with increased risk of some cancers, including skin cancer and lymphoma.

    Other risk factors:

    - Excessive UV exposure (sunbeds)
    - Skin type I (always burns, never tans)
    - Multiple moles
    - Family history and previous history of melanoma

03. **Types:**

    - Nodular melanoma
    - Lentigo melanoma
    - Acral lentiginous melanoma
    - Superficial spreading

04. **Prognosis:**

    - Recurrence of melanoma is determined by Breslow thickness
    - 5-year survival is based on the TNM classification

COMPLETE CDM KEY

Case 3: Eczema

01. **Pathophysiology:**
    - There is disruption of the epidermis due to underlying filaggrin protein defect
    - This exposes dermis immune cells to environmental antigens
    - There is an IgE antibody response which leads to an inflammatory response
    - Scratching further disturbs the epidermal barrier which leads to further inflammation

02. **Atopic eczema** is the most common type. It usually develops in early childhood and affects 20% of children under 12 years in the UK

03. **Management:**
    - General measures – avoid exacerbating factors (soap. Washing powder. Etc.)
    - Emollients, bath / soap alternatives (e.g. Hydromol)
    - Topical therapy – topical steroids
    - Oral therapies – antihistamines for itch, antibiotics / antivirals if superadded infection
    - Phototherapy and immunosuppressants for non-responsive patients

04. **Complications:**
    - Secondary bacterial infections (crusted weeping lesions)
    - Secondary viral infection. e.g. eczema herpeticum

COMPLETE CDM KEY

Case 4: Necrotising ffasciitis

01. In severe, rapidly spreading cellulitis, crepitus and systemic upset (fever, tachycardia), always consider necrotising fasciitis!

02. Most common causative organism = Group A haemolytic streptococcus

03. **Immediate management:**
    - Assess ABCDE
    - IV access and bloods including FBC, U&Es LFTs, CRP, blood cultures
    - ECG, ABG and CXR (look for other sources of infection)
    - X-ray soft tissues over infection site – the presence of anaerobes is responsible for the halimark finding of gas formation later in polymicrobial necrotising fasciitis
    - IV fluid resuscitation – patients will often be septic and in extremis (they may ultimately require inotropes)
    - Urinary catheter for fluid balance measurement
    - Analgesia – the affected area is exquisitely painful and tender (remember – if you have a patient that appears to have cellulitis but they are sdisproprotionately sore....... Think necrotizing fasciitis! If there is clinical doubt, you can use the laboratory Risk indicator for Necrotizing Fasciitis (LRINEC) score.
    - IV antibiotics (based on local guidelines)
    - Urgent referral for extensive surgical debridement.

CHAPTER

OBSTETRICS AND

GYNAECOLOGY

CASE 1

SCENARIO

COMPLETE CDM KEY

A 30-year-old woman presents at 31 weeks of gestation with suspected premature rupture of membranes.

01. Give 2 complications of ruptured membranes.

02. Your perform a speculum exam. What are you looking for and what investigations (if any) would you perform during the exam?

03. What would you monitor to try to identify the early onset of complications?

COMPLETE CDM KEY

The patient goes into labour and the baby is born. The paediatric team are in attendance.

04. What signs would indicate respiratory distress?

COMPLETE CDM KEY

OBSTETRICS AND GYNAECOLOGY

CASE 2

SCENARIO

A 27-year-old woman presents to A&E with a 6-over history of right iliac fossa pain and vaginal bleeding. Her last menstrual period was 8 weeks ago.

01. What is your differential diagnosis?

02. What specific questions would you want to know from the history?

03. List 2 investigations you would carry out.

COMPLETE CDM KEY

04. Name a treatment option for each of your differential diagnoses.

05. What should be given to a rhesus-negative woman who bleeds during pregnancy?

OBSTETRICS AND GYNAECOLOGY

CASE 3

SCENARIO

You see a 255-year-old primigravida in maternity triage. She is 31 weeks pregnant. She has been referred by here midwife with pedal oedema. Her blood pressure is 148/106mmHg and there is proteinuria (+) on urinalysis.

01. What is the likely diagnosis?

02. What 3 investigations would you order to assess the mother?

03. You arrange for an ultrasound. How could this help to assess the fetal condition?

COMPLETE CDM KEY

04. What other investigation would be useful?

05. The consultant is planning a caesarean section and asks you to prescribe the mother a steroid. How does the administration of steroids benefit the pre-term infant?

COMPLETE CDM KEY

OBSTETRICS AND GYNAECOLOGY

ANSWERS

Case 1: Premature rupture of membranes

01. **Complications:**

    - Premature labour
    - Infection (such as chorioamnionitis) – can cause fetal distress and death

02. **Specutum exam:**

    - Confirm ruptured membrance-looking for discharge at posterior fronix; test discharge with nitrazine paper (amniotic pH-7, vaginal pH-4); amniotic fluid also crystallises on drying whereas vaginal secretions do not
    - Look for signs of labour onset – cervical effacement, dilatation and show
    - Assess for infection with high vaginal swabs for microscopy, culture and sensitivity

03. **Observations:**

    - Temperature – pyrexia may indicate infection
    - Fetal heart rate – fetal tachycardia (HR>160bpm) may suggest infection
    - Uterine contractions – regular painful contractions (often assessed using cardiotocography (CTG) alongside cervical dilatation and effacement indicate preterm labour

04. **Respiratory distress:**

    - Progressing techypnoea
    - Increased respiratory effort with signs such as grunting. Nasal fiaring, intercostal recession, tracheal tug. Head nodding and cyanosis

COMPLETE CDM KEY

Case 2: Amenorrhoea and abdominal pain

01. **differential diagnosis – amenorrhoea, abdominal pain and PV bleeding:**
    - Ectopic pregnancy
    - Miscarriage

02. **History:**
    - Previous pregnancies – any history of ectopic pregnancy or miscarriage
    - Is she sexually active (and is she using contraception)?

03. **Investigations:**
    - Blood testing – FBC, U&Es, β-hCG, group and save
    - Transvaginal ultrasound (abdominal US is suboptimal)

04. **Management:**
    - Ectopic pregnancy – methotrexate or salpingectomy
    - Miscarriage – conservative / evacuation of retained products of conception

05. **Rhesus – negative mothers:** anti-D immunoglobulin – this is usually given around 30 weeks of gestation and again 72h after birth

Case 3: Pre-eclampsia

01. **Diagnosis:** Pre-eclampsia

02. **Bloods:**

    - Full blood count – low platelets in severe pre-eclampsia
    - Liver function tests – elevated LFTs in severe pre-eclampsia
    - Urea and electrolytes – creatinine elevated in severe pre-eclampsia

    It is important to recognize **HELP** syndrome which may develop from preeclampsia. HELLP- haemolysis, elevated LFTs, low Platelets.

03. **Ultrasound:**

    - Growth – abdominal circumference, femoral length; this allows comparison of any variation from normal and determination of intrauterine growth restriction (IUGR).
    - Assess umbilical artery using a Doppler ultrasound – informs of any placental blood flow resistance
    - Assess fetal movements – again contributes to the picture of biophysical wellbeing
    - Quantity the liquor volume – determines oligohydramnios or polyhydramnios which impacts fetal growth

04. **Fetal assessment:** cardiotocography (CTG)

05. **Steroids in prematurity:** steroids stimulate the production of surfactant in the lungs, encouraging maturation; lung prematurity can cause neonatal respiratory distress syndrome (associated with high mortality and morbidity) and giving steroids improves fetal survival.

CHAPTER

PAEDIATRICS

CASE 1

COMPLETE CDM KEY

SCENARIO

You are working a night shift in paediatrics when you are paged to review a baby boy who was born at term, 4 hours ago. Following examination, you think that the baby has Down syndrome.

01. What neurological sign is likely to be present?

02. The baby's parents are present. How would you give them the diagnosis?

COMPLETE CDM KEY

03. To confirm the diagnosis you organise some investigations. What is the most likely karyotype?

04. What type of karyotype would significantly increase the risk of his parents having another baby with Down syndrome?

Four weeks later the baby is taken to his GP with poor feeding. On exam, there is a loud pansystolic murmur but there is no cyanosis and all peripheral pulses are palpable.

05. What are you top 2 differential diagnosis for the causes of the murmur?

COMPLETE CDM KEY

COMPLETE CDM KEY

PAEDIATRICS

CASE 2

SCENARIO

An 8-month –old boy is brought to A&E by his worried mother. He has not been his normal self and he has passed "redcurrant jelly" stools in his nappy. You think this could be due to intussusception.

01. Briefly describe the pathophysiology of intussusception.

02. What 3 physical signs would you look for?

03. What 2 investigations would you use to support the diagnosis?

COMPLETE CDM KEY

04. List 3 complications of intussusception.

05. Give 1 possible definitive treatment.

COMPLETE CDM KEY

COMPLETE CDM KEY

PAEDIATRICS

CASE 3

SCENARIO

You are working in A&E when a 3-month-old boy is brought in by his parents. He is fitting in his mother's arms. His mother tells you that he has been generally unwell for 2 days. Today he had a high temperature. He has been fitting for 10 minutes.

01. What is the most likely diagnosis?

02. Before giving any pharmacological therapy, what is your immediate management plan?

COMPLETE CDM KEY

The child stops seizing. On re-assessment, he is much improved but looks miserable. There are no signs of meningitis and you are unable to find a source of infection.

03. You need to terminate the seizure. How do you achiever this?

_____

_____

04. What other investigation is needed?

_____

_____

05. After a period of observations, the child is discharged. What advice would you give to his parents to prevent this happening in the future?

_____

_____

_____

COMPLETE CDM KEY

06. What is the prognosis regarding future seizures?

COMPLETE CDM KEY

PAEDIATRICS

CASE 4

SCENARIO

A 6-week-old boy is brought to A&E with persistent vomiting. The vomiting started 8 days earlier and he always seems hungry after vomiting. The GP had diagnosed reflux and started him on Gaviscon. You do an ABG and the results are:

	Results	Reference range
pH	7.65	7.35- 7.45
PCO_2	5.0kPa	4.6-6.0kPa
PO_2	12.0kPa	10.0-13.5kPa
Base deficit	+5.8	0
HCO_3^-	33mmol/L	22-33mmol/L

01. You think the child looks dehydrated. List 5 ways to assess the degree of dehydration.

COMPLETE CDM KEY

02. Describe the abnormalities seen in the blood gas.

03. What is the most likely diagnosis?

04. Briefly describe now how these blood gas results arises.

05. On abdominal examination, there is a mass in the upper abdomen. What investigation will you order?

COMPLETE CDM KEY

06. If your diagnosis is confirmed, what operation is needed?

COMPLETE CDM KEY

PAEDIATRICS

CASE 5

SCENARIO

You see an 8-year-old boy in the ENT outpatient clinic. He complains of a 7-month history of blocked nose, recurrent sore throat, earache and poor hearing. The child has had multiple courses of antibiotics and decongestants.

01. What are your top 2 differential diagnoses?

02. Give 4 other features from the history that you would enquire about.

COMPLETE CDM KEY

03. Investigations reveal bilateral conductive hearing loss. What 2 surgical options may be indicated?

04. Briefly outline how the above treatment might improves his symptoms.

COMPLETE CDM KEY

PAEDIATRICS

CASE 6

SCENARIO

A 5-year-old girl presents to paediatric A&E with pain and swelling of her left knee.

01. What are your top 3 differential diagnoses?

_____

_____

_____

_____

_____

02. The child is very distressed and this makes clinical examination difficult. Give 2 methods which could help you to assess her pain.

_____

_____

_____

COMPLETE CDM KEY

03. She eventually calms down a little and allows you to examine her knee – give 3 features you would look for.

04. The registrar aspirates the knee. What 2 other investigations would you do?

COMPLETE CDM KEY

PAEDIATRICS

CASE 7

SCENARIO

You are FY2 doing a post in paediatrics. You spend the day completing newborn baby checks.

01. Why is it important to carry out baby checks prior to discharge?

02. Give 2 examples of clinical problems that may be identified during the routine baby check.

03. You are asked to perform a Guthrie test. How would you explain this to the parents?

COMPLETE CDM KEY

04. Give 2 conditions that are checked by the Guthrie test.

The hospital is part of interdisciplinary research collaboration. The consultant wants to include this child in an ongoing study.

05. What 4 principles would you discuss with the parents when seeking approval for patient participation?

COMPLETE CDM KEY

COMPLETE CDM KEY

PAEDIATRICS

CASE 8

SCENARIO

You assess a 3-month-old girl in A&E. she has been unwell for the last few hours with fever and vomiting. You think she needs a full septic screen.

01. What is the most reliable means of collecting an uncontaminated urine sample?

02. Give 2 other ways of obtaining a urine sample in paediatrics.

03. List 2 other components of the septic screen.

COMPLETE CDM KEY

04. What 2 criteria are used to define a laboratory culture diagnosis of UTI?

05. What is the most common causative organism?

06. The child is admitted and commenced on IV antibiotics. What treatment should she receive on discharge pending further investigation?

07. What radiological investigation would you request for follow-up?

PAEDIATRICS

CASE 9

SCENARIO

You are an FY2 carrying out routine baby checks. You examine a term baby at day 2 after birth and note mild jaundice. There are no other obvious abnormalities.

01. Why is it important to recognise jaundice in newborns?

02. Outline 2 specific types of jaundice that are most concerning and give reasons why.

COMPLETE CDM KEY

03. Give the treatment for neonatal jaundice and briefly outline its mechanism of action.

04. The baby improves and is ready for discharge. This is the mum's first child and she is anxious about going home. Outline community support that will be available to her.

COMPLETE CDM KEY

PAEDIATRICS

CASE 10

SCENARIO

You are reviewing a baby girl who is 6 months old. She was born by caesarean section at 32 weeks of gestation. She spent some time in NICU and required CPAP. Mum is concerned that her development is slightly delayed.

01. Give 4 developmental milestones you would expect her to be meeting.

02. What is the most likely cause for development delay in this case?

COMPLETE CDM KEY

03. Outline how you would explain this to her mother – what is the prognosis?

You discuss the importance of immunisations in preventing childhood illness. Mum saw on social media that there is a link between autism and MMR. After a long discussion, you have reassured here that immunisations are safe.

04. She asks when her child will receive her first and second MMR vaccinations.

COMPLETE CDM KEY

COMPLETE CDM KEY

PAEDIATRICS

CASE 11

SCENARIO

A 26-year-old mother who is 30 weeks pregnant attends maternity triage stating that her "waters have broken" and that her "baby is coming" you suspect she is in premature labour.

01. The parents are understandably anxious that their baby is going to be born prematurely. Name 3 complications of prematurity.

_____

_____

_____

_____

_____

_____

The baby girl is born by SVD. She is assessed by paediatrics who take her to NICU because she is showing signs of respiratory distress.

02. What 5 signs would you expect to see?

_____

_____

COMPLETE CDM KEY

03. What investigations would you order?

04. Give 4 treatments that you would consider in this case.

COMPLETE CDM KEY

PAEDIATRICS

CASE 12

SCENARIO

You are an FY2 in paediatrics doing baby checks. As you are examining a baby, the mother asks to talk to you about breastfeeding.

01. Give 5 benefits of breastfeeding for the baby.

02. Give 4 maternal benefits as a result of breastfeeding.

COMPLETE CDM KEY

03. The mother is worried that her baby is not feeding well. How would you handle this situation?

04. On discharge, the mother asks you how she will know her baby is getting enough milk. What will you advise?

COMPLETE CDM KEY

PAEDIATRICS

CASE 13

SCENARIO

You assess a 7-year-old boy in A&E. He had a viral upper respiratory tract infection last week and now presents with abdominal discomfort and feeling generally unwell.

On examination, he is interacting well and there are no signs of meningism. His abdomen is generally tender but there is no peritonism. You note a vasculitic-looking, non-blanching rash over his legs and buttocks. FBC, CRP and coagulation are normal.

01. What is your initial diagnosis?

02. What other symptoms may be present?

03. What is the underlying disease process?

COMPLETE CDM KEY

04. What other investigations will you carry out?

05. What is your management plan?

COMPLETE CDM KEY

PAEDIATRICS

CASE 14

SCENARIO

You are completing a baby check on a baby girl born at term. On examination you note swollen feet, a wide neck, significantly spaced nipples and you are unable to detect a femoral pulse. You ask your registrar for advice. He thinks that these features could be due to turner syndrome.

01. What investigation would you carry out to confirm the diagnosis and what results would you expect?

02. How would you deliver the news to the parents?

COMPLETE CDM KEY

03. List 3 other features you might see in Turner syndrome.

04. What other specially would you involve in this baby's care?

COMPLETE CDM KEY

COMPLETE CDM KEY

PAEDIATRICS

CASE 15

SCENARIO

You are asked to see a baby girl born 30 hours ago by SVD. Staff on the post-natal ward are concerned that she has not been feeding well. They handover that she is lethargic and the skin appears mottled. Respiratory rate is 50 but she is apyrexial.

01. The nurses are taking O_2 saturations, but what 2 other basic observations would you measure?

02. What 4 investigations would you perform?

03. Describe an investigation to the parents and explain the reasons for it.

COMPLETE CDM KEY

As you are assessing the baby girl, she continues to deteriorate. Oxygen saturations are now 72% on air. You commerce high flow oxygen but this does not improve the situation.

04. What is your diagnosis?

05. Why has the deterioration occurred?

Your consultant decides that this child required transfer to a tertiary center and referral on.

06. Which specialty should she be referred to?

COMPLETE CDM KEY

07. The parents are understandably incredibly concerned. The tertiary center is far away from their home and family. How do you justify the transfer?

PAEDIATRICS

ANSWERS

Case 1: Down syndrome

01. **Neurological feature in majority of babies with Down syndrome at birth:** hypotonia

02. **Breaking bad news:**
    - Setting – should be quiet and free of interruption; parents could bring friend or family for support
    - Perception – ask the parents what they understand so far
    - Invitation – how much information do the parents want?
    - Knowledge – give information without jargon or long complex monologues: pause for parents to digest and question
    - Empathise – recognise the parent's fragility at this time and offer what support you can
    - Strategy – inform parents of what the plan is, moving forward, than summarise and check understanding

    The SPIKES approach above is an effective template for approaching all difficult news delivery consultations.

03. **Karyotype:** trisomy 21

04. **Inheritance:** unbalanced translocation

05. **Acyanotic murmurs:**
    - Ventricular septal defect (VSD)
    - Patent ductus arteriosus (PDA)

COMPLETE CDM KEY

Both are acyanotic pansystolic murmurs that are seen often in Down syndrome patients.

Case 2: Intussusception

01. **intussusception:** a condition in which the bowel telescopes and a proximal portion of the bowel invaginates into a distal portion

02. **Signs:**

    - Bile-stained vomit and rectal bleeding (classically 'redcurrant jelly' stool)
    - Episodic intermittent inconsolable crying – child often sleeps between episodes
    - Sausage-shaped abdominal mass
    - Later in the disease process-signs of shock (tachycardia, hypotension)

03. **Investigations:**

    - Abdominal X-ray – looking for signs of obstruction
    - Abdominal ultrasound – looking for characteristic target sign (or doughnut sign) of intussusception

04. **Complications:**

    - Bowel ischaemia
    - Perforation and peritonitis
    - Shock

05. **Treatment – air insufflation:**

    - Air can be introduced into the bowel with a rectal catheter; the retrograde pressure is often enough to correct the intussusception and in children, most cases are resolved this way and surgery is not required.

Case 3: Febrile convulsions

01. **Diagnosis:** febrile convulsion

02. **Immediate management:**
    - ABCDE assessment, paying particular attention to airway management and oxygen sats
    - Check blood sugars
    - Observations – HR, RR, temperature
    - Gain IV access

03. **Drug treatment:** if IV access gained – IV lorazepam; otherwise buccal midazolam or rectal diazepam

04. **Fever in child under 3 months:** a septic screen is essential in this case-cultures of blood and urine should be taken; lumbar puncture should be performed and CSF sent for microscopy, culture and sensitivity.

05. **Preventing febrile convulsions:**
    - Manage fevers with paracetamol and ibuprofen, and cool child by stripping to pants/vest
    - Ensure child is vaccinated to prevent unnecessary infection with subsequent feverish episodes

06. **Prognosis:** children have a 1 in 3 chance of a second convulsion if they develop a fever in the future; there is no significant increase in risk of future epilepsy.

Case 4: Pyloric stenosis

01. **Assessing dehydration:**
    - Poor skin turgor
    - Decreased urine output
    - Dry mucous membranes
    - Prolonged capillary refill time
    - Pallor
    - Raised heart rate
    - Reduced consciousness

02. **Blood gas:** raised pH and bicarbonate confirms an alkalosis; PCO_2 is normal and there is a positive base excess consistent with a metabolic alkalosis (PO_2 is normal)

03. **Diagnosis:** Pyloric stenosis

04. **Pathophysiology of the blood gas in pyloric stenosis:** pyloric stenosis leads to vomiting which results in loss of hydrochloric acid from the stomach resulting in a metabolic alkalosis; there is subsequent renal compensation as bicarbonate reabsorption is maximised and the resulting picture is one of hypochloraemic metabolic alkalosis

05. **Investigation:** ultrasound scan of abdomen shows hypertrophy of pylorus

06. **Operation:** Ramstedt's pyloromyotomy

COMPLETE CDM KEY

Case 5: ENT

01. **Differential diagnosis:**
    - Otitis media with effusion
    - Recurrent tonsillitis

02. **History:**
    - Discharge from the ear- otitis media with effusion
    - Degree of hearing loss – if interfering with school / learning
    - Recurrent URTIs (such as sore throats and rhinorrhea) more in line with tonsillitis
    - Assess for systemic symptoms such as fever, poor feeding or lethargy which may indicate progression of illness requiring more urgent management
    - Also assess for complications associated with these differentials, such as vertigo, nystagmus, tinnitus, aural swelling and facial paralysis

03. **Surgical options:**
    - Insertion of grommets
    - Adenoidectomy

04. **Surgical improvement in symptoms:**
    - Grommets allow drainage of fluid from the middle ear which should reduce any pain and improve hearing
    - Adenoidectomy relieves obstruction and reduces future nasal congestion symptoms

COMPLETE CDM KEY

Case 6: Swollen knee

01. **Differential diagnosis:**
    - Septic arthritis
    - Reactive arthritis
    - Haemarthrosis, i.e. haemophilia

02. **Assessing pain:**
    - Use of pain rating scales such as sad faces increasing up to smiley faces (or any appropriate to developmental stage)
    - Evaluate child's behavior, taking cues from them and any physical changes as describe by caregiver

03. **Knee examination:**
    - Decreased range of movement (comparing with opposite side)
    - Any crepitus felt across the joint
    - Any changes in gait – assessing for antalgic gait and ability to weight bear

04. **Investigations:**
    - Blood test, including FBC, CRP, blood cultures and a coagulation screen
    - Imaging – X-ray of knee and hip

COMPLETE CDM KEY

Case 7: Baby check

01. **Purpose of baby checks:**
    - Detection of congenital abnormalities
    - Reassure caregiver(s) and provide opportunity for them to raise any concerns about their child

02. **Examples of congenital abnormalities that may be detected:** cleft palate, developmental dysplasia of the hip, imperforate anus, cardiac murmurs and cataracts

03. **Explaining the Guthrie test:** a routine test performed in all babies at 5-7 days after birth which involves taking a small amount of blood from the baby's heel which is then tested in the lab; it is used to detect common and serious disease that are important to pick up early.

04. **Guthrie tests for:** sickle cell disease, cystic fibrosis, congenital hypothyroidism, metabolic disease such as phenylketonuria.

05. **Ethics in research:**
    - Autonomy – it is their right to decide yes or no and the decision will not impact care moving forward
    - Benefit of research – will improve medical practice in the future
    - Confidentially – details will not be disclosed beyond the scope of the research
    - Informed consent – can only test for research purposes with parental consent, and the purpose of the research and any risk must be disclosed; there will likely be no benefit to the baby

COMPLETE CDM KEY

Case 8: Septic screen

01. **Specimen type:** suprapubic aspirate

02. **Urinalysis:**
    - Clean catch midstream sample of urine
    - Catheter specimen of urine

03. **Investigations:**
    - Bloods – FBC, U&Es, CRP, cultures
    - Lumbar puncture
    - Lactate

04. **Laboratory definition of UTI:**
    - Any bacteria in suprapubic aspirate
    - $>10^5$ organisms per ml of fresh urine

05. **Most common causative organism:** *E.coli*

06. **Prophylactic antibiotics:** evidence for the use of prophylactic antibiotics is deficient, but a prophylactic does should be considered until the initial urinary tract imaging has been completed

07. **Imaging:** ultrasound scan of bladder and renal tract

Case 9: Paediatric jaundice

01. **Important to recognise jaundice because:**
    - High levels of conjugated bilirubin may lead to kernicterus
    - Jaundice may be secondary to underlying disease such as haemolysis or infection

02. **Worrying jaundice:**
    - Jaundice occurring <24h after birth is always abnormal; causes include sepsis, rhesus haemolytic disease, ABO incompatibility and red blood cell abnormality
    - Prolonged jaundice (lasting > 14days) indicates ongoing disease such as hypothyroidism, cystic fibrosis and biliary atresia

03. **Treatment:** phototherapy is a method of delivering blue/green UV light to the skin where it is able to break down bilirubin and alleviate jaundice

04. **Community support:**
    - Community midwife – mothers can phone to ask for help or advice regarding their new baby; the community midwife will also carry out a routine check – up at day 10 to ensure that mother and baby are well
    - GP-available to help with any health concerns in both short and long term
    - Social services-can help with financial and housing services, and they can also be contacted if there are any concerns regarding wellbeing.
    - Support groups- many communities have 'new mum' networks for mothers to together with their children and share advice / stories; these are proven to have a positive impact on maternal mental health

COMPLETE CDM KEY

Case 10: Development milestones

01. **6 month milestones:**
    - Sitting up without support
    - Palmar grasp
    - Monosyllabic sounds (such as "ma", "da", "ba")
    - Puts food in mouth

02. **Likely cause for delayed milestones:** prematurity – catch –up development is needed

03. **Explanation of delayed milestones in prematurity:**

    Because she was born early, she requires some more time to develop to the level of her peers who have had more time in utero to mature; the prognosis is good and she is likely to catch up with her peers within the next year and certainly be on par with them by 2 years of age

04. **Immunisations:**
    - First MMR vaccination is at 12 months
    - Second MMR vaccination is at 3 years

COMPLETE CDM KEY

Case 11: Premature birth

01. **Complications of prematurity:**

    - Underdevelopment of the lungs - may lead to respiratory distress syndrome due to lack of surfactant
    - Difficulty feeding due to GI tract immaturity and a poorly developed suckling reflex; jaundice may also result from underdeveloped GI tract failing to metabolise bilirubin
    - Hypothermia due to lack of body fat and underdevelopment of the skin leading to poor temperature control; incubator may be required
    - Ventricular haemorrhage is not uncommon in babies <34 weeks due to failure of blood vessels to cope with pressure shifts – these children may go on to develop learning difficulties or cerebral palsy

02. **Signs of respiratory distress:** tachypnea (>60 breaths/min), apnoea (at end stage), cyanosis, intercostal / subcostal recession, expiratory grunting, nasal flaring

03. **Investigations:** FBC, chest X-ray, ABG, pulse oximetry

04. **Management:**

    - General supportive care – warming / incubator
    - Supplementary O_2 – may require CPAP or invasive ventilation
    - Surfactant via endotracheal tube
    - Antibiotics until pneumonia / infection can be excluded

COMPLETE CDM KEY

Case 12: Breastfeeding

01. **Benefits to the baby:**

    - Decreased infant mortality rate
    - Lower risk of gastrointestinal infection
    - Sharing of maternal immunoglobulins and and lymphocytes means the the child is less likely to be infected by pathogens to which mum has been exposed
    - Otitis media and pneumonia are much rarer in breastfed children
    - Breastfed children are at much lower risk for autoimmune disease and food allergies
    - Breastfed children are shown to have slightly greater IQs then their non-breastfed peers

02. **Maternal benefits:**

    - Can help mother lose pregnancy – related weight gain
    - Works as a natural contraceptive; known as the lactational amenorrhoea method (LAM) – out of 100 women who use LAM during the first 6 months following childbirth, 1-2 of them may become pregnant. Women should not rely on this method of contraception once they introduce solid food to their baby.
    - Enhances mother to baby bonding (improving mother's mental health)
    - Breastfeeding is inexpensive and natural
    - Breastfeeding when done promptly following birth induces contraction of the uterus to a smaller size and therefore minimizes post-partum haemorrhage

03. **Poor feeding?**

    - Reassure mum and encourage her to persist
    - Assess her feeding technique
    - Exam child's suckling reflex with your finger (also assessing for cleft palate)
    - Examine the child for any obvious abnormality prohibiting good feeding behavior

COMPLETE CDM KEY

04. **Is breastfeeding going well?**

- Feeds per day – day 0-1 = at least 4; day 2+ = at least 8
- Length of feeds – between 5 and 40 minutes (if consistently > 45 min may mean baby is not feeding effectively)
- Wet napples – day 1- at least 2; day 2= at least 3; day 5= at least 6

COMPLETE CDM KEY

Case 13: Non – blanching rash

01. **Diagnosis – abdominal pain and purpuric rash (in absence of meningism):** Henoch – schonlein purpura (HSP) – triad of purpura, arthritis and abdominal pain

02. **Other symptoms:**
    - Arthritis / arthralgia
    - PR bleeding
    - Haematuria
    - Scrotal pain or swelling

03. **HSP caused by:** immune – mediated vasculitis (IgA) affecting capillaries, arterioles and venules

04. **Investigations:**
    - Urinalysis with microscopy and culture
    - Abdominal ultrasound scan – intussusception may occur in these patients
    - Urea and electrolytes to assess kidney function

05. **Management:**
    - Reassure parents that this is generally a benign and self-limiting illness
    - Provide analgesia (paracetamol and ibuprofen) to manage abdominal and joint pains
    - IV fluids should be considered and kidney function monitored
    - Oral steroids may be commenced, but this should be discussed with a senior or a specialist first

COMPLETE CDM KEY

Case 14: Turner syndrome

01. **Investigation:** karyotyping should be carried out by geneticists; for Turner syndrome we would expect karyotyping to show an X chromosome monosomy (45XO) but if this is inconclusive, fluorescent in situ hybridisation (FISH) analysis may be carried out to confirm

02. **Breaking bad news:**

    SPIKES criteria are highly effective in difficult consultations:

    - **S**etting – should be quiet and free of interruption; parents could bring friend or family for support
    - **P**erception – ask the parents what they understand so far
    - **I**nvitation – how much information do the parents want?
    - **K**nowledge- give information without jargon or long complex monlogues; pause for parents to digest and question
    - **E**mpathise – recognise the parents' fragility at this time and offer what support you can
    - **S**trategy – inform parents of what the plan is. Moving forward, then summarise and check understanding

03. **Other features of Turner syndrome:** short stature, cubitus valgus (wide carrying angle), ptosis, nystagmus, downward-sloping eyes, rudimentary gonads, cardiac defects (echo should be carried out), shield – shaped chest, poor social skills and multiple melanocytic naevi

04. **Referral:** cardiology referral should be made due to the impalpable femoral pulse – this is a sign of coarctation of the aorta – a congenital defect common to Turner's; an endocrine referral may be required in future due to pubertal delay or growth restriction

Case 15: Mottled newborn

01. **Observations:**

- Heart rate
- Blood pressure
- Respiratory rate (already given)

02. **Investigations:** FBC, ABG, chest X-ray and echocardiogram

03. **Explain an investigation:**
    - Echocardiogram – 'heart ultrasound' that allows visualisation of the heart and assessment in real time which can tell us how well the heart is functioning
    - ABG – blood test usually taken from the wrist. Blood is taken from and artery rather then a vein. The test allows us to assess how well the lungs are performing and gives us an insight into how much oxygen and carbon dioxide in the blood and can help us direct treatment
    - FBC – full blood count. This is a blood test that allows us to test for anaemia or raised white cells that can occur in infection and other conditions.
    - CXR – a chest X-ray allows us to look at the lungs and the outline of the heart. It can give an indication of infections such as pneumonia.

04. **Diagnosis:** duct – dependent cyanotic heart disease – consider this in infants that are cyanotic, with signs of shock (mottled) and who don't improve with supplemental oxygen.

05. **Deterioration due to:** closure of the duct following delivery

06. **Will require input from:** paediatric cardiology

07. **Tertiary referral:**

COMPLETE CDM KEY

- Their child most likely has a congenital heart problem that is best dealt with by a specialist team with experience and skill sets in this field
- Deterioration with saturations of 74% suggest she required immediate input by doctors who manage such conditions regularly

COMPLETE CDM KEY

CHAPTER

PSYCHIATRY

CASE 1

SCENARIO

A 28-year-old man is brought into A&E after taking an overdose of amitriptyline.

COMPLETE CDM KEY

01. What toxic effect of amitriptyline would you be worried about and how would you investigate this?

02. What features from the history would be indicative of serious suicidal intent?

03. What is the most important aspect of the risk assessment to consider?

COMPLETE CDM KEY

04. Give 3 psychiatric disorders most associated with suicide risk.

PSYCHIATRY

CASE 2

SCENARIO

A 46-year-old woman presents to her GP with low mood. Further history elicits that she is drinking heavily.

01. What would you ask from the history to assess the severity of her alcohol problem?

The GP takes bloods.

02. What would you expect to see on a blood film?

03. What would you ask in the history to assess whether she was dependent on alcohol?

COMPLETE CDM KEY

Chronic alcohol abuse can have detrimental effects on the cardiovascular, neurological and gastrointestinal systems.

04. Give one chronic adverse effect for each system above.

COMPLETE CDM KEY

COMPLETE CDM KEY

PSYCHIATRY

CASE 3

SCENARIO

A 29-year-old homosexual man presents to the GP with symptoms of anxiety. He says he constantly worries that he will contract HIV. He smells strongly of antiseptic and when questioned, admits that he washes his hands up to 30 times each day.

01. What are these symptoms?

02. Give 5 characteristic features of such symptoms.

COMPLETE CDM KEY

03. Give you top 2 differential diagnoses.

04. What neurotransmitter is most often associated with these symptoms?

05. Which drug treatment is most effective?

COMPLETE CDM KEY

COMPLETE CDM KEY

PSYCHIATRY

CASE 4

SCENARIO

You are an FY2 in general practice. A 29-year-old man comes to see you with stress. He has recently broken up with his girlfriend and is struggling at work. Throughout the consultation he stares at the flood and has poor eye contact.

01. List 4 differential diagnoses of depression.

02. Give 2 biological symptoms of depression.

You have a long discussion with him and explain that you would like to start an antidepressant.

COMPLETE CDM KEY

03. What 2 groups of antidepressant could be used and what are their respective mechanisms of action?

_____

_____

_____

_____

_____

_____

Two weeks later the patient is admitted to hospital after an attempted suicide. His father found him unconscious at home surrounded by packets of co-condamol. On examination he has pinpoint pupil and GCS of 8.

04. What two drugs would you administer?

_____

_____

COMPLETE CDM KEY

05. What other complications can develop later and should be anticipated?

COMPLETE CDM KEY

PSYCHIATRY

CASE 5

SCENARIO

A 22-year-old nurse has recently been diagnosed with schizophrenia and has started taking chlorpromazine. Four days later he complains of a stiff neck and jerking movements of his face and tongue.

01. What is the name given to this side – effect?

02. Outline the drug mechanism that leads to this side – effect and say where in the brain it originates.

03. Give 3 other side – effects caused by the same drug mechanism.

COMPLETE CDM KEY

04. How would you treat these side – effects?

05. Give 2 examples of antipsychotic drugs that are less likely to cause these side – effects.

COMPLETE CDM KEY

PSYCHIATRY

CASE 6

SCENARIO

A 19-year-old woman is brought to A&E 3 hours after taking a mixed overdose including paracetamol, diazepam, herbal sleeping tablets and amitriptyline. She smells strongly of alcohol and she tells you she has drunk 2L of cidr. She appears breathless. With oxygen saturations of 85% on air. Her heart rate is 120bpm and she is normotensive. You think you can hear right basal crepitations.

01. The FY 1 has ordered a chest X-ray and paracetamol levels. What other investigations will you request?

COMPLETE CDM KEY

02. The chest X-ray shows opacification of the right lung base. What is the most likely diagnosis and how will you manage this?

03. Paracetamol level comes back high (120mg/L at 4h). How will you manage this?

04. Over the next 2 hours, the patient deteriorates, and you move her to resus. She has become less responsive with a GCS of 6. What will you do?

COMPLETE CDM KEY

COMPLETE CDM KEY

PSYCHIATRY

CASE 7

SCENARIO

A 22-year-old student has been brought to the University health service by his friends. They are concerned by recent odd behavior. He has been wandering around campus claiming to be the son of God.

01. List 4 of Schneider's first rank symptoms of schizophrenia.

02. What risk factor for developing schizophrenia should you think about in a university student?

03. Various neurotransmitters have been implicated in mental illness. Give 2 examples of dopamine pathways n the brain.

COMPLETE CDM KEY

Your patient is prescribed an antipsychotic. Four months later, he presents to his GP with a tremor in his hand.

04. What has caused this? Give 2 other clinical signs that may be seen.

The patient's father is understandably very concerned. He had high hopes that his son would be the first in the family to graduate form University

05. He asks you what the chances of this happening are?

COMPLETE CDM KEY

Unfortunately, your patient doesn't respond to first-line treatment and the psychiatrist starts clozapine.

06. What regular investigations need to be carried out and why?

PSYCHIATRY

ANSWERS

Case 1: Amitriptyline overdose

01. **Amitriptyline:** amitriptyline toxicity can lead to ventricular arrhythmias which should be assessed using ECG monitoring

02. **Risk assessment:**
    - If there is evidence of planning
    - If help was sought after the act
    - If there were ' final acts' – leaving notes, cancelling bills, writing a will
    - If there is any regret over suicide's failure

03. **Most important aspect:** continued risk to the patient – does the patient still wish to kill themselves?

04. **Psychiatric conditions and suicide risk:**
    - Depression
    - Schizophrenia
    - Post – traumatic stress disorder
    - Substance use disorder
    - Eating disorder
    - Personality disorder

COMPLETE CDM KEY

Case 2: Alcohol abuse

01. **Assessing alcohol behaviour:**

    - **Drinking behaviours** – quantity of alcohol consumed and over how may days per week? Does the patient think of alcohol when they first wake in the morning? Has their drinking repertoire narrowed?
    - **Patient feelings** – does patient feel they should cut back? Have they ever felt guilt over drinking so much?
    - **Impact on life** – does the patient feel that alcohol has impacted their relationship or work life?

02. **Blood film in alcoholics:** macrocytosis (raised MCV)

03. **Assessing dependency:**

    - High tolerance
    - Compulsion to consume alcohol
    - Continued use despite evidence of harm
    - Withdrawal symptoms
    - Neglect of other tasks/ interests
    - Narrowing of repertoire

04. **Adverse effects:**

    - Cardiovascular system – dilated cardiomyopathy, arrhythmias, hypertension
    - Nervous system – memory disturbance, cortical atrophy, Korsakoff's psychosis ± Wernicke's encephalopathy
    - Gastrointestinal system – oesophageal varices, pancreatitis, hepatitis, cirrhosis, haemorrhoids

Case 3: Repetitive behaviors

01. **Symptoms:** obsessive thoughts and compulsive actions

COMPLETE CDM KEY

02. **Symptoms of obsessive thoughts and compulsive actions:**
    - Recurrent
    - Cause anxiety / stress / fear
    - Intrusive to function
    - Patient has insight
    - Completing ritual may alleviate some stress
    - Resistance may worsen anxiety

03. **Differential:**
    - Obsessive compulsive disorder (OCD)
    - Generalised anxiety disorder

04. **Neurotransmitter in OCD:** serotonin (5-HT)

05. **Treatment:** SSRI, e.g. fluoxetine, sertraline

COMPLETE CDM KEY

Case 4: Depression

01. **Differential diagnosis of depression:**

    - Substance misuse
    - Dementia
    - Hypothyroidism
    - Schizophrenia
    - Anaemia
    - Adjustment reaction

02. **Biological Symptoms:**

    - Loss of appetite
    - Insomnia

03. **Antidepressant and mechanism of action:**

    - **SSRI** – stops the reuptake of serotonin in the synapse leading to increased serotonin duration in the synapse increased serotonin activity)
    - **SNRI** - stop the reuptake of both serotonin and noradrenaline, prolonging their tie in the synapse
    - **MAOI** – inhibits the enzymes responsible for reuptake of neurotransmitters

04. **Co-codamol overdose – reduced GCS and pinpoint pupils:**

    - Naloxone – opiate antagonist
    - N-acetylcysteine (Parvolex) prevents paracetamol – induced hepatotoxicity by replenishing glutathione stores

05. **Complications:**

    - Liver and kidney failure may follow due to paracetamol overdose
    - Coagulopathy and multi-organ failure are possibilities

Case 5: Antipsychotics

01. **Side – effect:**

    - Acute dystonic reaction – an extrapyramidal side-effect (abnormal face and body movements) and dyskinesia, which occur more commonly in children or young adults and appear after only a few doses
    - Tardive dyskinesia (rhythmic, involuntary movements of tongue, face and jaw), which usually develops on long-term therapy or with high dosage, but it may develop on short-term treatment with low doses-dosage, but it may develop on short-term treatment with low doses-short-lived tardive dyskinesia may occur after withdrawal of the drug.

02. **Mechanism of dystonia:** this reaction results from excessive dopamine (D2) receptor antagonism in the basal ganglia of the brain

03. **Other antipsychotic side – effects:**

    - Parkinsonism
    - Hypotension
    - Akathisia (motor restlessness)

04. **Managing acute dystonia;**

    - Withdraw prochiorperazine and initiate an atypical antipsychotic
    - IM procyclidine – initiate an antimuscarinic to counteract these side-effects

05. **Atypical antipsychotics:**

    - Olanzapine
    - Quetiapine
    - Risperidone

Case 6: Overdose

01. **Investigations:**
    - Urea & electrolytes
    - Liver function test
    - Arterial blood
    - Glucose
    - Full blood count
    - INR
    - ECG should **<u>always</u>** be performed in tricyclic overdose

02. **Overdose (reduced GCS) + reduced sats + chest signs =** likely aspiration pneumonia which should be treated with amoxicillin and metronidazole; if there is penicillin allergy, swap amxoicillin for clarithromycin

03. **Treatment of paracemtamol overdose:** *N*-acetylcysteine (Parvolex. NAC) IV is the treatment of choice because it can prevent paracetamol – induced hepatotoxicity if given within the first 8h of the overdose (it may also be effective up to and possibly beyond 24h).

04. **Management of acute deterioration:**
    - Repeat ABCDE assessment
    - Repeat observations. ABG bloods and ECG
    - Call for senior help and contact ITU as airway may be at risk – consider airway adjuncts.

Case 7: Schizophrenia

01. **Schneider's first rank symptoms:**
    - Auditory hallucination s
    - Thought broadcast
    - Thought insertion / withdrawal / interruption
    - Somatic hallucinations
    - Delusional perception
    - Believing actions / feelings are controlled by external source

02. **Potential schizophrenia risk in this case:** smoking cannabis

03. **Dopamine pathways:**
    - Nigrostriatal
    - Mesolimbic
    - Tubero-infundibular
    - Mesocorticolimbic

04. **Side-effect-dyskinesia / tremor:** this is an extrapyramidal side-effect associated with dopamine antagonism in the nigrostriatal pathway; other signs include parkinsonism, dystonia, akathisia and tardive dyskinesia

05. **Prognosis:** the course of schizophrenia is variable: in general 25% will have one acute event then recover, 25% will have recurrent acute events, 25% will have chronic illness starting with an acute event, and 25% will have chronic illness starting insidiously.

06. **Clozapine monitoring:** FBC – assessing for neutropenia as a sing of agranulocytosis

COMPLETE CDM KEY

PRACTICE PAPER

CASE 1

SCENARIO

A 49-year-old woman attends the breast clinic after discovering a lump in her left breast. She is understandably worried because her mother died from breast cancer.

01. What examination features would you look for that would suggest breast cancer?

COMPLETE CDM KEY

02. In relation to breast cancer screening, what are the 3 components of triple assessment?

03. Name 3 key pieces of pathological information which will help determine prognosis following breast cancer surgery.

COMPLETE CDM KEY

04. She is prescribed letrozole; how does this drug work?

COMPLETE CDM KEY

PRACTICE PAPER

CASE 2

SCENARIO

A 19-year-old man is brought to A&E after being in a road traffic accident. He had to be removed from the car by the fire service. His heart rate is 125bpm and his blood pressure is 77/42mmHg. On examination you find bruising over the left side of his pelvis. You find blood at the external urethral meatus and suspect a fractured pelvis.

01. Apart from fracture, give 2 other injuries that could cause hypotension in this man.

02. Why is there blood at the external urethral meatus? To confirm your clinical suspicion, what examination would you perform?

COMPLETE CDM KEY

03. What X-ray would you consider for any major trauma patient?

04. The patient remain hypotensive. What would you do to treat the uncontrolled haemorrhage in this patient? Describe two treatment options.

05. What is the overall mortality rate associated with this injury? List 2 causes of death.

COMPLETE CDM KEY

COMPLETE CDM KEY

PRACTICE PAPER

CASE 3

SCENARIO

An obese 76-year-old woman presents with a history of increasing pain in her right knee. She denies any other joint pains and she has no relevant past medical history.

01. What is the most likely diagnosis?

02. Give 2 features from her history that you would ask about to assess the severity of her symptoms.

03. Give 4 examination features you would look for to support you diagnosis.

COMPLETE CDM KEY

04. How would you medically manage this patient?

COMPLETE CDM KEY

PRACTICE PAPER

CASE 4

SCENARIO

A 70-year-old man complains of severe abdominal pain. His temperature is 38.4°C, heart rate is 130bpm and he has a raised WCC.

01. What clinical entity does the above scenario represent?

When you examine him, you find localised peritonism in the left iliac fossa.

02. What are your top 3 differential diagnoses?

COMPLETE CDM KEY

03. What is your immediate management plan?

04. What single investigation would you order to confirm the diagnoses?

The man continues to deteriorate despite maximal medial therapy. He is taken to theatre and laparotomy indicates that the sigmoid colon is the source of the peritonitis.

05. What surgical procedure may be indicated in this case?

06. Describe 2 pathological features of the most likely diagnosis.

_____

___

_____

___

PRACTICE PAPER

CASE 5

SCENARIO

A 62-year-old woman presents with sudden onset of a red and painful right eye. Her history rules out a foreign body or trauma as the cause.

01. List 4 further questions you would ask to help with you differential diagnosis.

02. After inspecting the eye and examination of the pupil you evaluate her vision. Give 2 tests you would use and briefly describe how each test in carried out.

COMPLETE CDM KEY

Examination reveals corneal oedema, a fixed dilated vertically oval pupil, the absence of a red reflex and a shallow anterior chamber.

03. Name the most likely diagnosis.

04. Earlier in the day, the patient had attended thhe diabetic clinic. What iatrogenic factor could have contribute to her acute problem?

COMPLETE CDM KEY

05. What should you do next?

COMPLETE CDM KEY

PRACTICE PAPER

CASE 6

SCENARIO

A 54-year-old man attends your surgery complaining of worsening cough. Over the past 4 years he has had an intermittent cough, but he is now producing a greater volume of phlegm than usual and says that he struggles when walking upstairs. He has smoked 40 cigarettes per day for 30 years.

You arrange spirometry and the results are as follows:

	Predicate	Observed	Post-dilator
FVC (L)	4.78	2.05	2.12
FEV_1, (L)	3.66	0.55	0.59
TLC (L)	7.01	8.63	
RC/TLC (%)	31	68	
$DL_\%$ (ml/min/Hg)	26	20	

01. Give 2 parameters that predict lung function in a normal, non-smoking patient.

02. What spirometry pattern is demonstrated in this patient? Describe 2 further features indicated by the results.

Page | 378

COMPLETE CDM KEY

03. After arranging for some baseline blood tests, results show a raised haemoglobin of 19.9g/dl. What is the physiological explanation for the raised haemoglobin?

04. You discuss the need to stop smoking with the patient. Name 3 methods of smoking cessation you could discuss.

COMPLETE CDM KEY

COMPLETE CDM KEY

PRACTICE PAPER

CASE 7

SCENARIO

A 27-year-old woman delivered her first child via spontaneous vaginal delivery 2 hours ago. Nursing staff inform you that she is passing a large volume of PV blood and looks very pale.

01. Give 4 major causes of post-partum haemorrhage.

02. How would you manage the bleeding?

COMPLETE CDM KEY

03. Give 4 risk factors for post – partum haemorrhage.

PRACTICE PAPER

CASE 8

SCENARIO

Whilst completing a rotation in general practice, a 15-year-old girl comes to see you complaining of acne.

01. Name 3 types of acne.

02. List 4 initial treatment options for acne.

COMPLETE CDM KEY

Following multiple treatment attempts, she is still suffering from acne. Dermatology have recommended starting isotretinoin therapy.

03. What information should you give to her before starting this?

04. What 2 tests would you carry out prior to commencing treatment?

COMPLETE CDM KEY

COMPLETE CDM KEY

PRACTICE PAPER

CASE 9

SCENARIO

During a newborn baby check, you assess a child's hips and hear a loud clunk on hip movement.

01. Which 2 techniques would you use to assess the hips in a newborn baby check?

02. Give 2 risk factors for developmental dysplasia of the hip (DDH).

03. Outline the management of DDH.

04. Why is it important to identify DDH?

COMPLETE CDM KEY

COMPLETE CDM KEY

PRACTICE PAPER

CASE 10

SCENARIO

A 54-year-old woman attends your GP surgery following regular episodes of reflux over the past 2 weeks.

01. Name 3 tests that could be used to check for H. pylori.

02. How would you treat H. pylori?

COMPLETE CDM KEY

This patient's initial H.pylori test was negative.

03. What other options are available for managing gastro-oesophageal reflux disease?

   _____

   _____

   _____

   _____

   _____

   _____

04. Why is it important to manage reflux?

   _____

   _____

   _____

COMPLETE CDM KEY

COMPLETE CDM KEY

PRACTICE PAPER

ANSWERS

Case 1:

01. **Clinical features of breast cancer:**

    - Massage – often tethered to underlying tissue and non-smooth in texture
    - Skin features such as peau d'orange appearance
    - Nipple inversion
    - Bloody nipple discharge
    - Palpable axillary lymph nodes
    - Systemic features e.g. weight loss and malaise

02. **Triple testing:**

    - Breast examination
    - Imaging – ultrasound in women <35 years and mammongram for women >35 years, due to breast density changes associated with ageing
    - Tissue biopsy – usually core biopsy, but occasionally fine – needle biopsy

03. **Prognosis following breast cancer surgery:**

    - The Nottingham prognostic index:
        - Size of initial tumour
        - Number of nodes involved
        - Grade of the tumour

04. **Letrozole mechanism of action:** letrozole is an aromatase inhibitor which inhibits the enzyme aromatase form producing oestrogen

COMPLETE CDM KEY

Case 2:

01. **Haemorrhage in trauma:**
    - **Intraperitoneal haemorrhage** due to torn mesenteric vessels (sometimes iliac) or spleen / liver rupture
    - **Retroperitoneal haemorrhage** e.g. from rupture of aorta / IVC
    - Open wounds

02. **Blood at the urethral meatus in trauma:**
    - Pelvic displacement leads to an unstable pelvic fracture causing damage to urethra.
    - Examination
        - PR exam – feel for a high riding prostate
        - CT $\pm$ retrograde urethrogram

03. **Bedside imaging:**
    - Cervical spine X-ray
    - Chest X-ray (erect if possible)

04. **Management:**
    - Resuscitation – ABCDE approach with focus on fluid resuscitation and blood transfusion
    - Surgery by pelvic fixation – external fixation / open reduction and internal fixation with plates / screws
    - Interventional radiology to selectively embolise haemorrhaging vessel
    - Conservative – pelvic sling (bedsheet) / brace and supportive treatment, e.g. IV fluids blood

05. **Mortality:**
    - 10 – 20%
    - Hypovolaemic shock (due to uncontrollable haemorrhage)
    - Sepsis
    - Multi-organ system failure

Case 3:

COMPLETE CDM KEY

01. **Diagnosis:** osteoarthritis (right knee)

02. **History:**
    - Impact on daily living / mobility
    - Any pain at rest
    - Joint stiffness
    - Duration of morning stiffness
    - Any attempts to manage pain and their effectiveness

03. **Examination:**
    - Crepitus
    - Decreased range of movement
    - Joint instability
    - Muscle wasting
    - Joint tenderness
    - Joint effusions

04. **Medical management:**
    - Analgesia, e.g. NSAIDs, (caution in elderly)
    - Increase movement – exercise, physiotherapy, keeping active
    - Decreased load – lose weight, walking aids, supportive footwear

COMPLETE CDM KEY

Case 4:

01. **Clinical entity:**
    - Systemic inflammatory response syndrome (SIRS) – needs to fulfil at least 2 of the following criteria
        - Temperature <36 or > 38 °C
        - HR >90bpm
        - RR> 20
        - WCC > 12 or <4 x 10^9/L

02. **Differential diagnosis LIF pain:**
    - Diverticulitis
    - Perforated colon cancer
    - Inflammatory bowel disease

03. **Management:**
    - ABCDE
    - Oxygen therapy via a trauma mask
    - Gain IV access, take bloods (FBC, CRP, LFTs, U&Es, cross-match) and cultures: IV antibiotics and IV fluids
    - Analgesia: paracetamol for fever; morphine and consider anti-emetic

04. **Radiological investigation:** abdominal CT

05. **Surgery:** Hartmann's procedure: temporary colostomy and partial colectomy

06. **Pathological features in diverticulitis:**
    - Thickened muscular layer
    - Herniations of mucosa and submucosa through the muscularis externa

COMPLETE CDM KEY

Case 5:

01. **History:**
    - Has anything like this happened in the past? Any other past medical history (think associated conditions, i.e. connective tissue disorders/ autoimmune)?
    - Any history of intermittent blurring or haloes?
    - Photophobia – have your eyes become more sensitive to light?
    - Visual acuity – have you noticed a worsening of your vision?

02. **Test:**
    - Visual acuity test:
        - Using a snellen chart, have the patient stand 6m away with one eye covered at a time and ask them to read the smallest row of latters possible
    - Confronational visual field test:
        - Sit in front of the patient and ask them to cover one eye with their hand while covering you own eye for comparison
        - Move your fingers, starting peripherally and moving centrally until the patient can see them.

03. **Diagnosis:** acute closed – angel glaucoma

04. **Possible iatrogenic cause:** fundoscopy: being examined in a dark room, medication (anticholinergics, sympathetic agonists)

05. **Management:**
    - This is an ophthalmic emergency
    - Pilocarpine drops and acetazolamide
    - Urgent referral to ophthalmology department (will need to be admitted to hospital)

Case 6:

01. **Spirometry based on:**

- Height
- Age
- Weight

02. **Spirometry:**

    - Obstructive pattern
    - FEV_1 is reduced more than FVC
    - TLC is raised (may be indicative of emphysema)
    - Very mild post-dilator improvement
    - DL_{co} is reduced

03. **Polycythaemia:**

    - Chronic hypoxia leads to an increase in the production of erythropoietin (EPO)
    - This leads to an increase in erythropoiesis, resulting in polycythaemia

04. **Smoking cessation:**

    - Nicotine replacement therapies such as patches or chewing gum
    - Varenicline (Champix) is a medication that reduces nicotine cravings
    - Bupropion is a poorly understood medication proven to be effective in smoking cessation
    - E-cigarettes can be used as a step-down method that allows patients to have nicotine without the harmful effects of inhaling smoke

COMPLETE CDM KEY

Case 7:

01. **Post-partum haemorrhage – 4Ts:**

    - **Tissue** – placental tissue remaining in the uterus can stop contraction and constriction of blood vessels allowing haemorrhage which is why assessment of the placenta is so important
    - **Tone** – poor uterine tone means that blood vessels are not contracted against to stem blood flow
    - **Thrombin** – coagulopathies
    - **Trauma** – to the uterus during delivery can also lead to high volume blood loss

02. **Managing post-partum bleeding:**

    - Uterine massage to encourage uterine contraction
    - Medications to encourage uterine tone such as oxytocin and prostaglandins
    - Administration of blood products (including any required to correct clotting abnormalities)
    - Encourage infant suckling to help stimulate endogenous oxytocin production
    - Possible theatre attendance to remove any retained tissue or manage a site of injury

03. **Risk factors:**

    - Coagulopathy
    - High parity
    - Multiple pregnancies
    - Large baby
    - Poor surgical practice
    - Antepartum haemorrhage
    - Placenta praevia

Case 8:

01. **Acne:**

- Papulopustular
- Nodulocystic
- Comedonal

02. **Treatment:**

- Benzoyl peroxide cream
- Oral contraceptive pill (e.g. dianette)
- Antibiotics (e.g. lymecycline)
- Topical retinoids
- Photodynamic therapy

03. **Isotretinoin:**

- Isotretinoin is highly teratogenic and it is therefore very important that she takes all precautions to prevent becoming pregnant while on this drug
- She should also be informed of possible drops in her mood and impact on her mental health; if this becomes an issue, she should contact a GP
- Her skin and eyes may feel drier than normal but these are expected side-effects; if they become unmanageable she should get in touch with GP.

04. **Before commencing isotretinoin:**

- Pregnancy testing (β-hCG)
- LFTs (should be checked at each visit because they can become deranged)

COMPLETE CDM KEY

Case 9:

01. **Neonatal hip examination:**

    - Barlow test – dislocatable hip
    - Ortolani test – relocatable dislocation

02. **Risk factors:**

    - Breech birth
    - Family history
    - Oligohydramnios
    - Race (less common in black population)
    - Female
    - First born

03. **Management:**

    Management of DDH is largely about maintaining the femoral head within the acetabulum. Unsurprisingly, the earlier this can be done, the better the outcomes tend to be. If subluxation persists beyond 2 weeks, these children should have the joint reduced by being placed in a Pavlik harness to ensure correct joint placement. This is assessed using ultrasound. Harnesses are generally used for 6 weeks on a full-time basis, then reduced as per guidance of pediatricians

04. **Importance of identifying DDH:**

    If DDH is not detected, the femoral head does not rest in the acetabulum and the joint begins to close over, making it non-viable for reduction with a pavlik harness. Children with later diagnoses have poorer results and will probably require surgery to correct joint abnormality. This has associated risk and can require future surgery into adulthood

COMPLETE CDM KEY

Case 10:

01. ***H. pylori* investigations**

    - Urea breath testing
    - Faecal antigen testing
    - Serology (blood) testing

02. **Triple therapy:**

    - Omeprazole 20mg BD for 1 week
    - Clarithromycin 500mg BD for 1 week
    - Amoxicillin 1g BD for 1 week

03. **Further management:**

    - Lifestyle advice such as weight loss, smoking cessation, alcohol reduction and avoiding acidic foods
    - Ranitidine and other H_2 receptor antihistamines
    - Proton pump inhibitor s
    - Alginates
    - Nissen fundoplication
    - Highly selective vagotomy

04. **Untreated gastro-oesophageal reflux:**

    Presence of gastric acid in the oesophagus can lead to dysplastic changes / Barrett's oesophagus which in turn may lead to oesophageal carcinoma.

REFERENCES

Dr. Katharine et.al 2022 Canadian Medical Association-guidelines.

Conard Fischer et.al 2022 Master the boards 2 and 3 edition 2022

MRCP Part 1 El-Zohry MRCP Questions Bank 2013 1 st Edition.

Yusuf El-Zohry: mrcp-part-1-el-zohry-mrcp-questions-bank-2013-1-st-edition

MRCP Part 1 El-Zohry MRCP Questions Bank 2013 1 st Edition

Mastering the medical examination Paul M-2023

Khalid:Firstmrcp-part-1-el-zohry-mrcp-questions-bank-2013-1-st-edition

Crush Step 3 CCS: The Ultimate USMLE Step 3 CCS Review

Crush-step-3-ccs:-the-ultimate-usmle-step-3-ccs-review

COMPLETE CDM KEY

TORONTO NOTES 2022 Comprehensive medical reference and review for the Medical Council of Canada Qualifying Exam (MCCQE) Part I and the United States Medical Licensing Exam (USMLE) Step II 36th Edition Editors-in-Chief

Toronto-notes-2020-comprehensive-medical-reference-and-review-for-the-medical-council-of-canada-qualifying-exam-(mccqe)-part-i-and-the-united-states-medical-licensing-exam-(usmle)-step-ii-36th-edition-editors-in-chief

Clinical Decision Making (CDM) Sample Questions CASE1

Clinical-decision-making-(cdm)-sample-questions-case1

GUIDELINES FOR THE DEVELOPMENT OF KEY FEATURE PROBLEMS & TEST CASES

guidelines-for-the-development-of-key-feature-problems-&-test-cases

Clinical Decision Making (CDM) Sample Questions CASE1

Clinical-decision-making-(cdm)-sample-questions-case1

High Yield Surgery Shelf Exam Review

COMPLETE CDM KEY

High-yield-surgery-shelf-exam-review

PLAB 1700 Solved (no explanation)

Plab-1700-solved-(no-explanation)

~APLA~ MEDICAL Step 2 Cl&It

EdiUo ~apla~-medical-step-2-cl&It

The MRCP PACES Handbook, Second Edition

Samuel Blows: the-mrcp-paces-handbook,-second-edition

PASSMEDICINE NOTES GENERAL CONTENTS

Passmedicine-notes-general-contents

Crush Step 3 CCS: The Ultimate USMLE Step 3 CCS Review

Crush-step-3-ccs:-the-ultimate-usmle-step-3-ccs-review

COMPLETE CDM KEY

www.ingramcontent.com/pod-product-compliance
Lightning Source LLC
Chambersburg PA
CBHW020624220526
45464CB00001B/17